To Air Is Human

A guide for people with chronic lung disease (COPD)

Published and distributed by:
Pritchett & Hull Associates, Inc.

This book should not replace the advice or treatment your doctor gives you. It is to add to what you are already learning about chronic lung disease.

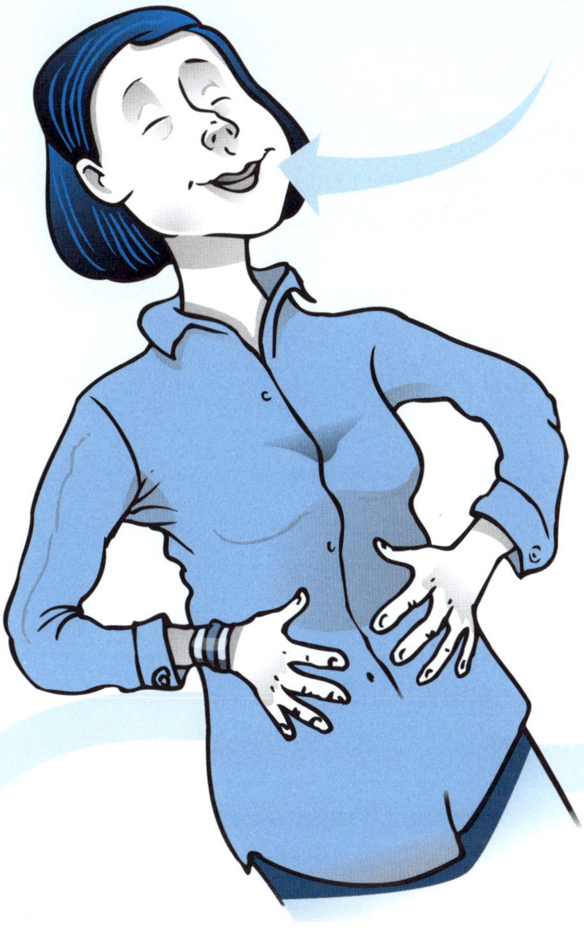

What's in this book

Chapter 1

How to Get Control of Your Breathing

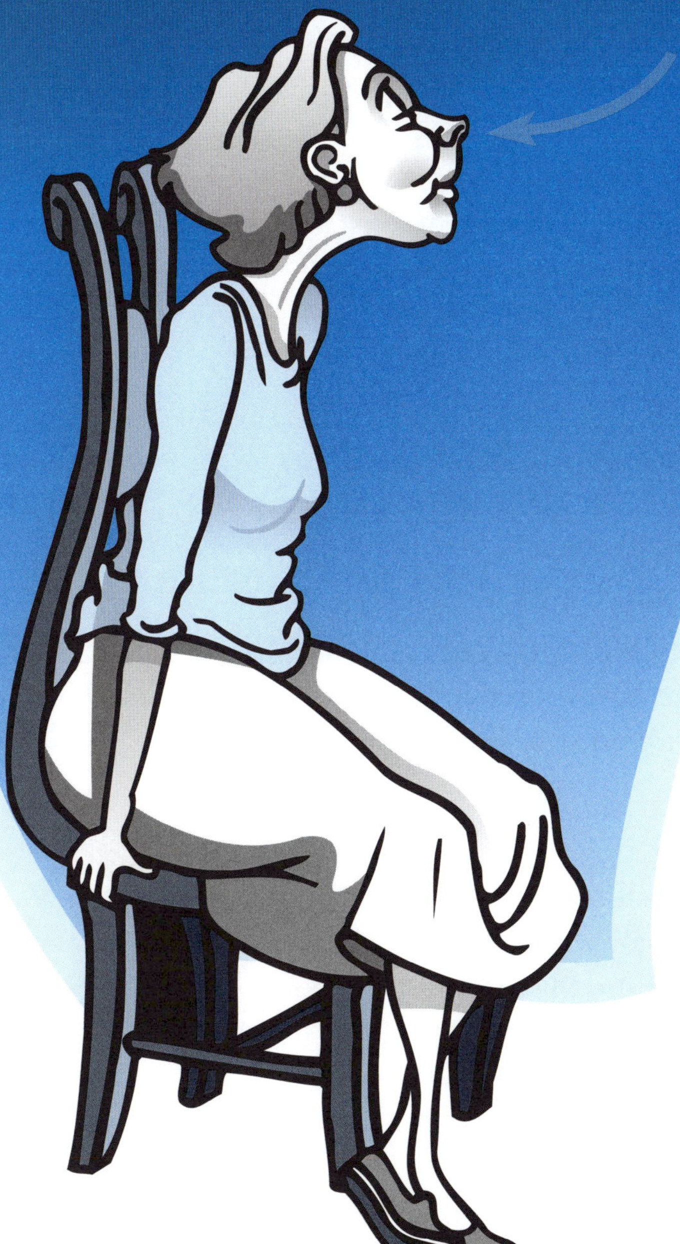

When you can't breathe

When you have COPD, many things can trigger shortness of breath. It is important to know ways to deal with it so that you can get through these difficult times. If you start to feel short of breath, don't panic. Follow these steps:

1. Stop and rest in **one** of the following positions:

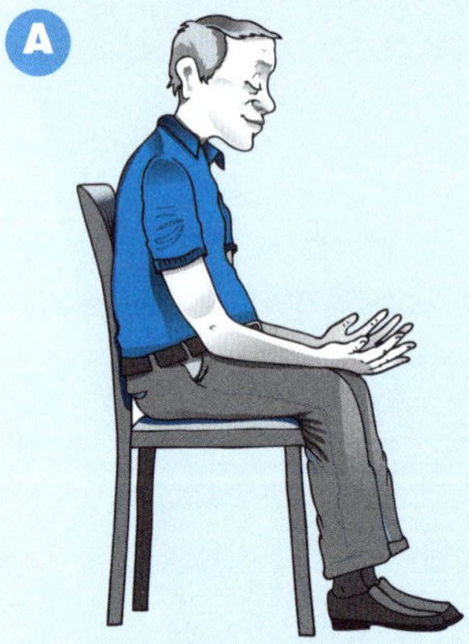

or

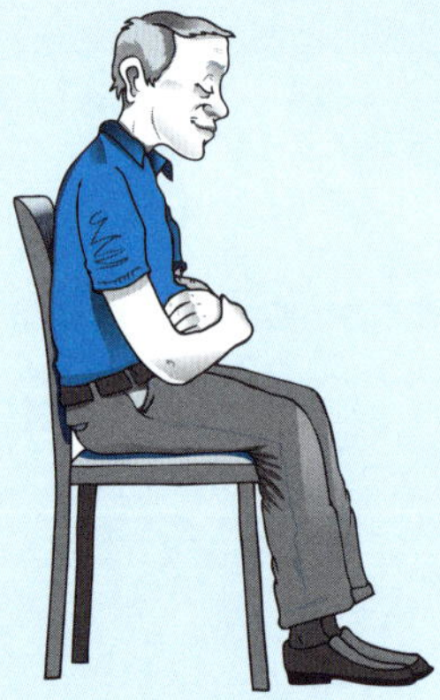

Sit with your feet on the floor and your back against the back of a chair. Roll your head forward, relax your shoulders and keep your knees rolled outward. Rest your arms and hands on your thighs, with your palms facing up ***or*** rest your hands on your stomach. (Do not lean on your hands.)

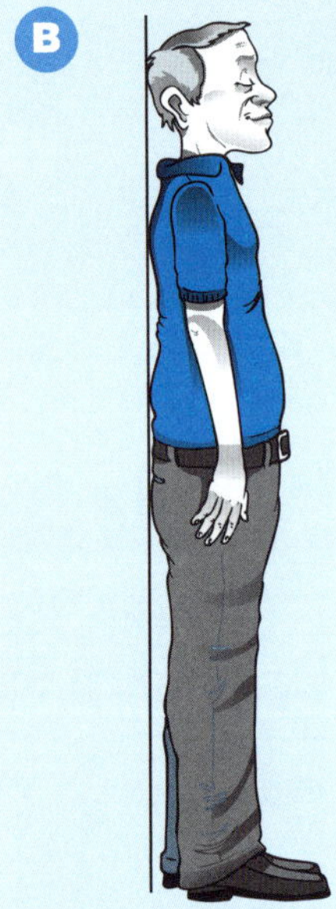

* **Stand** with your back against a hard surface such as a wall or pole. Stand with your feet slightly apart (away from the wall) and relax your head and shoulders.

Pull a chair close to a table. **Sit** in the chair with your feet on the floor and place a pillow on the table. Fold and rest your arms on the pillow, then lay your head on your arms.

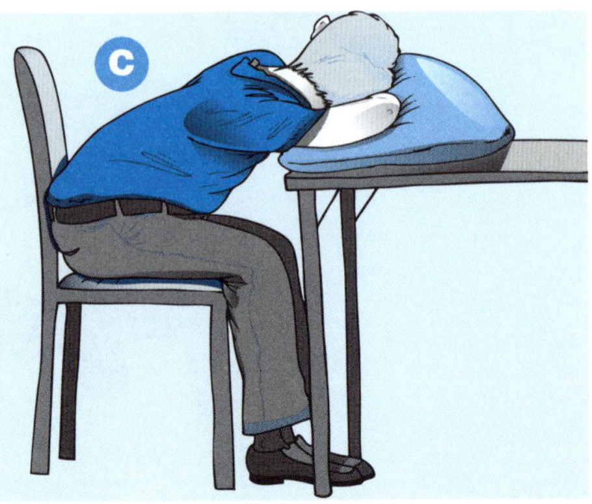

**If this position is too hard for you, try this: face the wall, stand with your feet slightly apart, place your forearms on the wall, then lean on your forearms for support.*

2. Breathe **in through your nose** and **out through your mouth** while trying to slow your breathing down. The slower you breathe, the more oxygen you can get into your body.

3. Use pursed lip breathing if it helps (see pages 6–7).

4. Begin to slow your breathing and breathe through your nose.

5. Begin diaphragmatic breathing (see pages 20–22).

6. Stay in this position for another 5 minutes or until you can breathe comfortably again.

Controlling stress

No matter what causes your shortness of breath, stress makes it worse. When you can't breathe, it is normal to become anxious. Your muscles become tense and need more oxygen. This causes you to breathe faster, work harder to take in more oxygen and feel even more anxious. This cycle makes it harder to control your breathing.

When you feel short of breath, do your best to relax and control your breathing. Practice pursed lip and diaphragmatic breathing when you're not short of breath so you will be ready to use these techniques when you need them. If you are prepared when shortness of breath occurs, you will get through it more smoothly and with less anxiety.

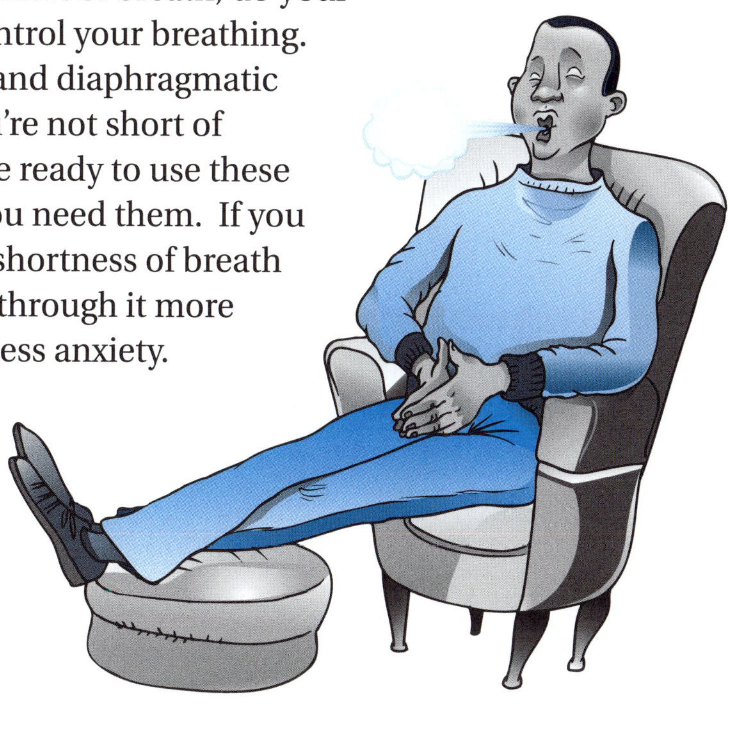

Controlled breathing

An important part of living with COPD is being able to control your breathing. The following types of controlled breathing will help you deal with shortness of breath and the anxiety it can cause. Ask your doctor to show you which of the following methods are right for you.

Pursed lip breathing

Pursed lip breathing helps get trapped, stale air out of your lungs. When you have COPD, your lungs are better at taking air in than letting air out. Stale air gets trapped in your lungs, keeping fresh air out. When this happens, you feel tightness in your chest or shortness of breath. Breathing faster will not bring you relief. Breathing out slowly through pursed lips will.

Practice pursed lip breathing every day. You may be too panicked to believe something as simple as pursed lip breathing can help, but it will.

Make this a habit. Do it several times a day when it's easy. Try doing pursed lip breathing before you take your inhaler, during your coffee break or when you're watching TV. Use pursed lip breathing during daily activities that make you short of breath. These may include bathing, cleaning the house, yard work or exercising.

Don't wait until you are in a breathing crisis to learn how to breathe more slowly.

How to do pursed lip breathing

Pursed lip breathing helps you when you find it hard to breathe. Learn this now so you won't panic when you feel short of breath:

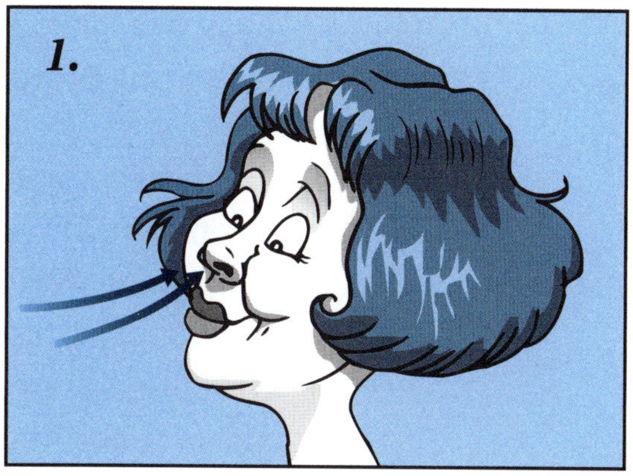

1. Breathe in slowly through your nose for 2 counts.

2. Purse your lips as if you were going to whistle.

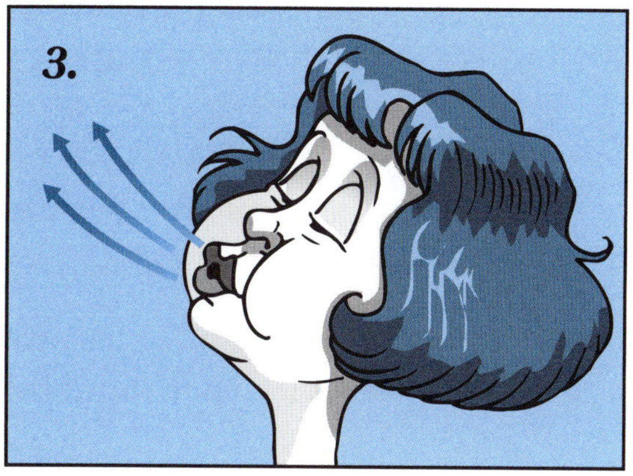

3. Breathe out gently through pursed lips for 4 slow counts. (Exhale twice as slowly as you inhale.) Let the air escape naturally.

4. Keep doing pursed lip breathing until you are not short of breath.

Breathing slowly this way can be done anywhere and at any time.

If you feel weak or tired when you need to do pursed lip breathing, first:

- sit upright in a chair with your hands on the sides of the chair (but don't put your weight on your hands)
- lean forward to shift your chest's weight forward

When you are wheezing

1. Do **pursed lip breathing** (pages 6–7). As you gently exhale through pursed lips, your airways stay open and air flows out more easily.

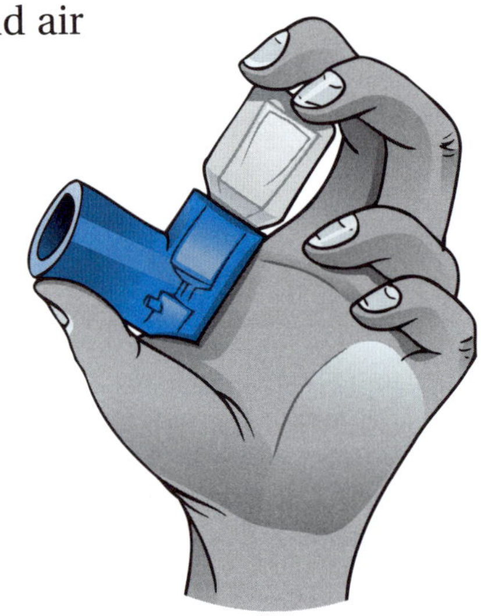

2. Take your **prescribed bronchodilator** (pages 39–42). Bronchodilators relax the muscles around your airways so they open up.

3. **Keep drinking fluids—** 8 to 16 cups a day (if allowed).

Wheezing is the noise you hear when exhaled air whistles through partly blocked air tubes (bronchi). You may wheeze because:

- The muscles around your air tubes squeeze in when something irritates them (asthma).
- You have too much mucus in your airways (bronchitis).
- Sometimes, when people have emphysema, the small airways in the lungs have collapsed.
- If your body tends to "hold water," the lining of your airways may swell. (This swelling may also be caused by infection or irritation.) This may also cause a "wet sound."
- The lining of your bronchial tubes is inflamed.

Coughing up mucus

Moving extra mucus out of your lungs is a key step in helping you breathe better. These techniques will help you do this.

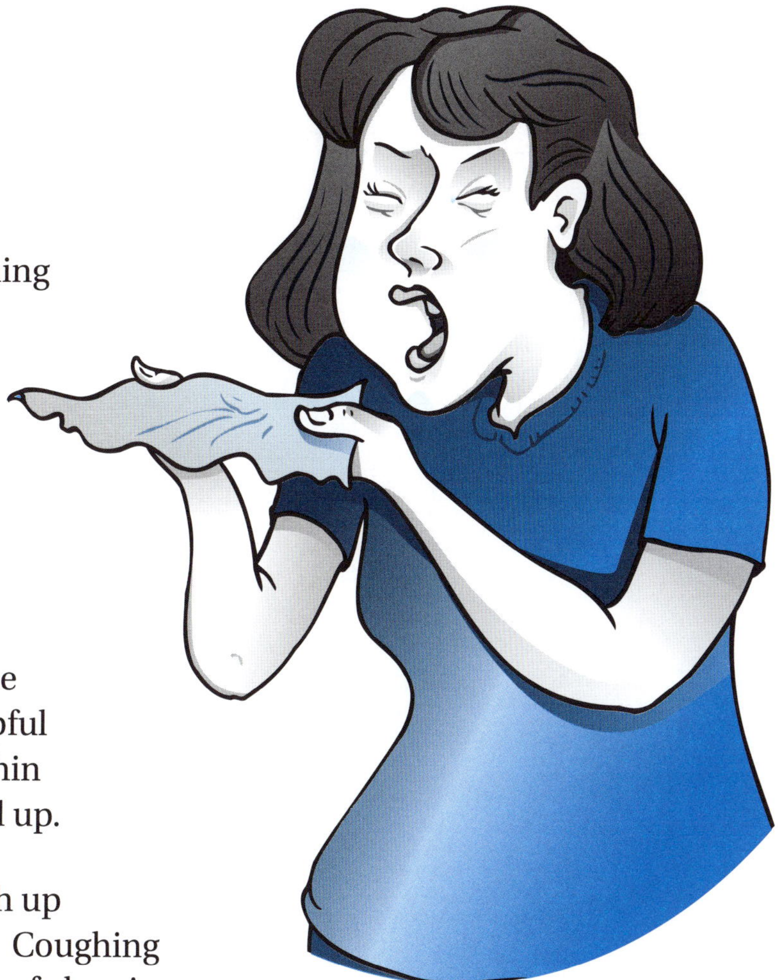

Controlled coughing

Controlled coughing (planned coughing sessions) can help you get the mucus out of your lungs. Plan these short sessions of coughing when you are rested and are not having coughing spells. These sessions are most helpful when your mucus is thin enough to be coughed up.

You need to cough up mucus when you can. Coughing is one of nature's ways of cleaning the lungs. Each day your lungs make extra mucus in response to "dirt particles" from smoke, pollution or germs you may inhale. If you don't get rid of extra mucus, you increase your chances of having shortness of breath, wheezing, infections or plugged airways.

How to do controlled coughing

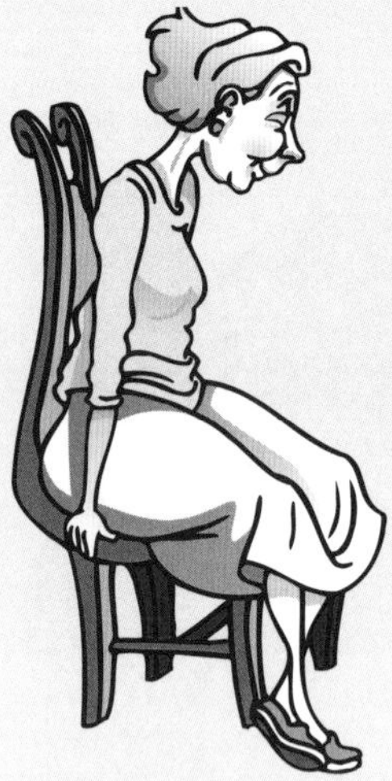

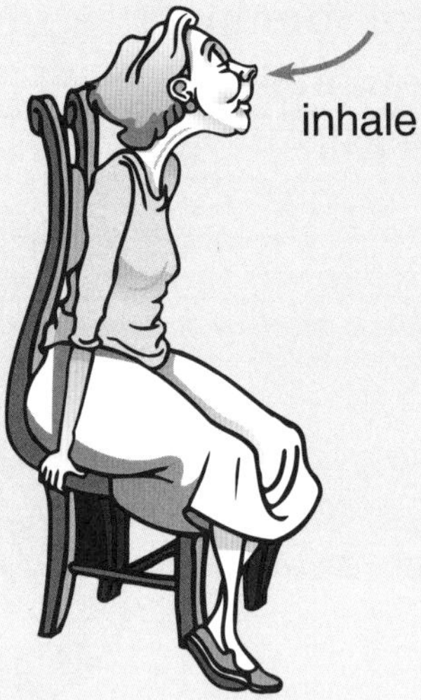

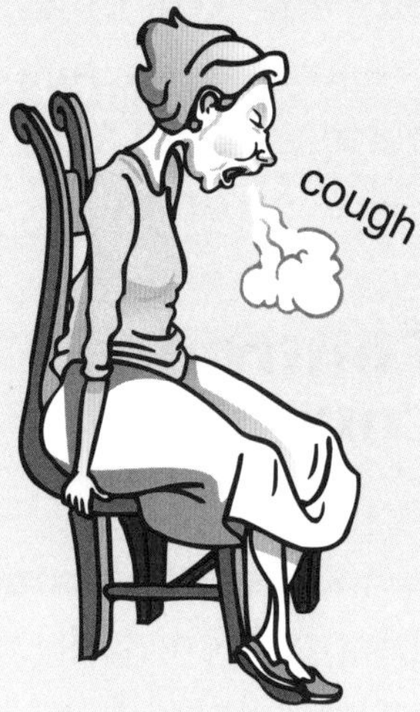

1. Sit up, and lean your head forward slightly.

2. Take a deep, slow breath through your nose and hold it for 2 seconds.

3. Cough once (to loosen mucus). Cough a second time (to move mucus forward). Try not to inhale between the 1st and 2nd cough. If you must, inhale **very slowly** and **not too deeply,** so you don't breathe the mucus back into your lungs.

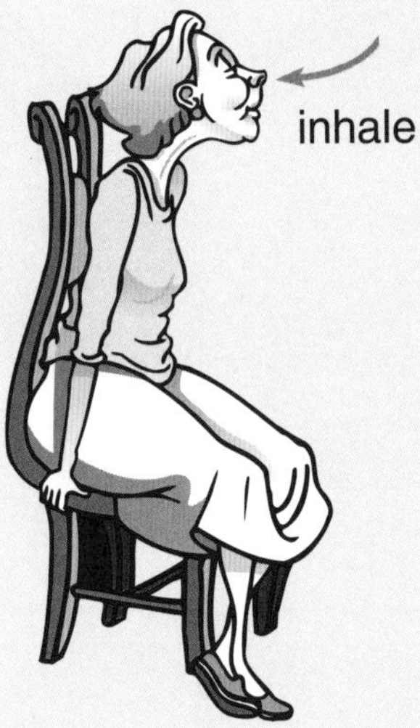

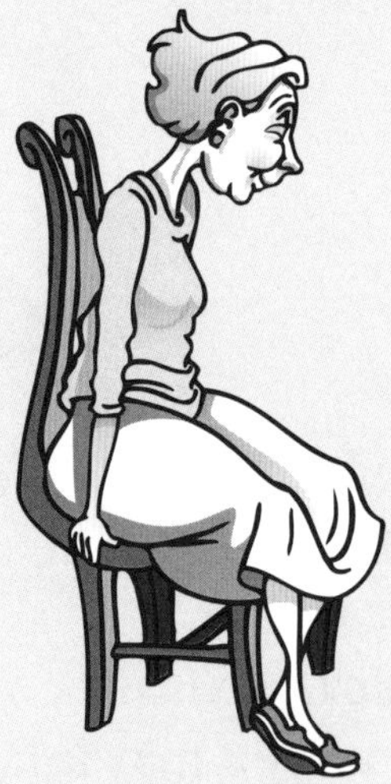

4. Wait a few seconds. Gently inhale. (A big breath may push mucus back into your lungs and make you cough again.)

5. Relax.

6. **Repeat these steps if you still need to cough.**

7. Spit coughed up mucus into a tissue and throw away.

> Do controlled coughing with **small, short coughs.** Avoid large blasts of air.

Water drinking

One of the most important treatments for lung disease is to drink a lot of water or other non-caffeinated fluids each day. Fluids keep mucus thin so it can be coughed up and out.

A buildup of thick, sticky mucus in the lungs is a main cause of shortness of breath, wheezing or dry, hacking coughs. Thick mucus is also a breeding ground for infection.

It may take a few days to a week or so of drinking a lot of fluids to notice a change in mucus. For most people, this means drinking 8–16 cups of water and other fluids a day.* At high altitudes (over 5,000 feet) or on long plane trips, even more water is needed. This much fluid will make you urinate more, but in time your body will adjust.

You can drink juice as part of your 8–16 cups, but count calories if you are trying to control your weight. To keep from feeling bloated, don't drink more than 1–2 glasses of fluid per hour, don't drink from a straw and don't drink a lot close to mealtime.

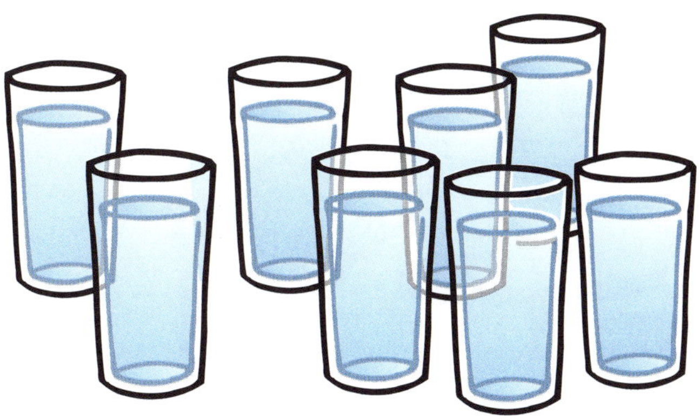

** Ask your doctor if 8–16 cups of fluid a day is OK for you. Some people can't drink a lot of fluids because of kidney disease, prostate trouble or heart disease.*

Don't drink a lot of colas, tea or coffee with caffeine. These make the body lose water and can cause you to feel nervous and "jittery." Small amounts of drinks with caffeine may be OK—2 to 4 cups a day. Some people with asthma find coffee or tea helps relieve wheezing at times.

Avoid alcoholic drinks. They can make it harder to cough. This promotes infections.

Don't use antihistamines, diuretics ("water pills") or cough suppressants unless your doctor tells you to take them for some other problem. These drugs dry the body out and make your mucus thicker. **Water is the best expectorant (cough producer).** Expectorants, other than water or other liquids, are rarely prescribed for someone with chronic lung disease.

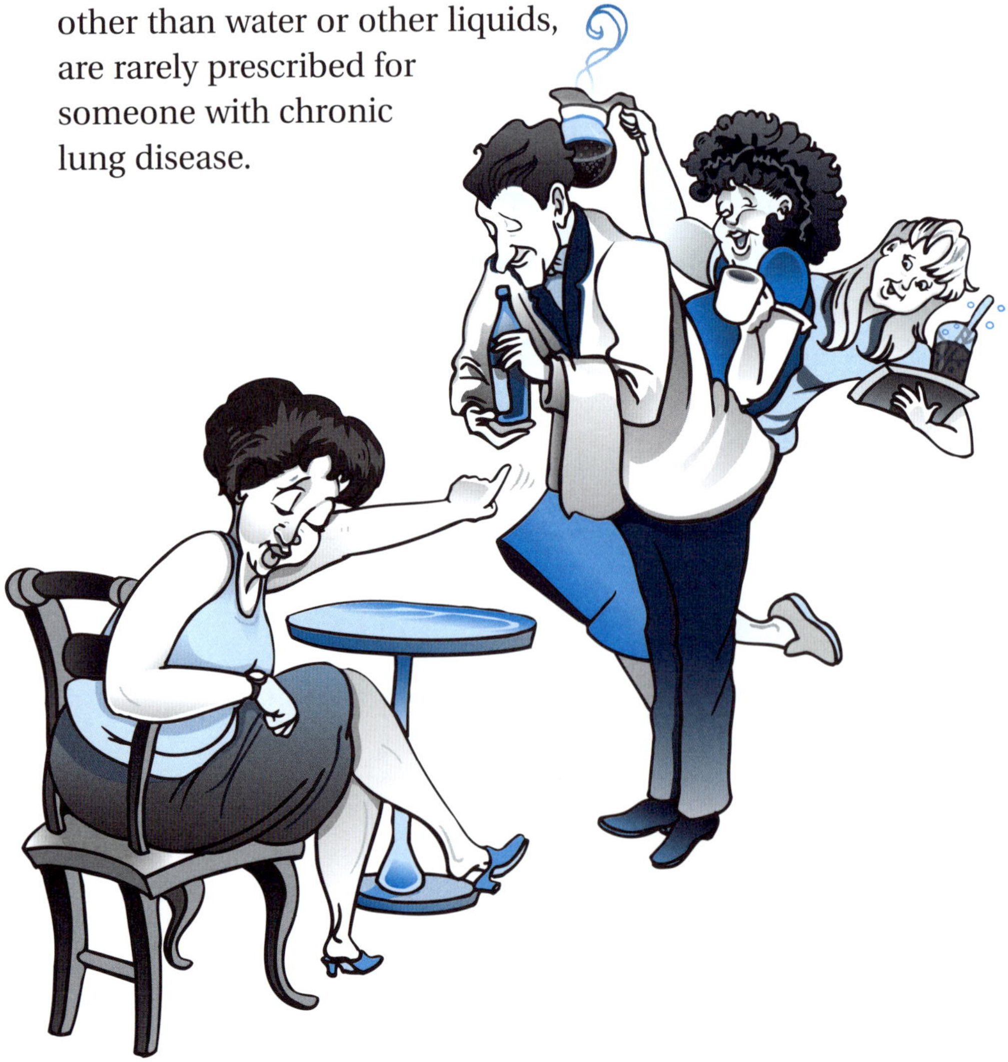

Infections

Infections can be serious when you have COPD. When mucus pools in the lungs too long, it gets thick and sticky and can become infected. It is important for you to know the warning signs of an infection:

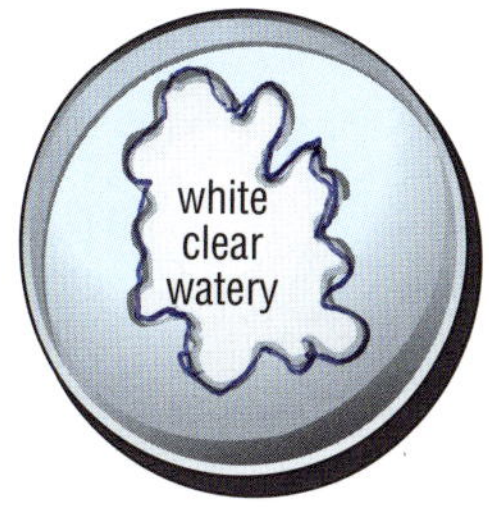

Healthy mucus

- an unusual increase or decrease in the amount of mucus
- an unusual increase in the stickiness of the mucus
- a change in the color of mucus—from clear or white to brown, yellow or green—or blood streaked mucus (Drinking lots of fluid, if allowed, and doing controlled coughing will help you bring up mucus so you can check it.)

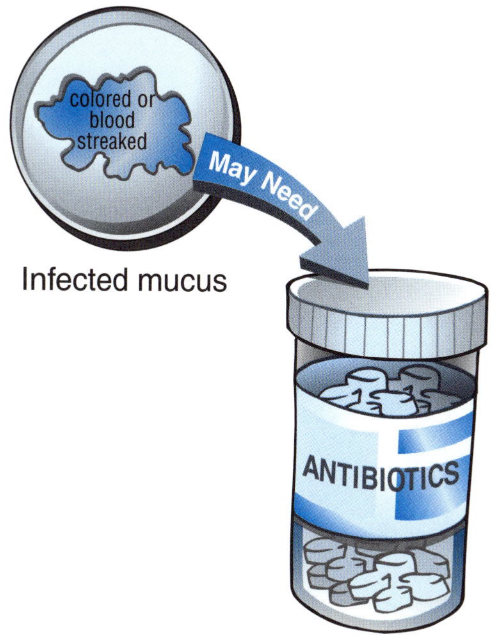

Infected mucus

- an unusual increase in shortness of breath
- swelling of your ankles
- a sudden increase or decrease in weight
- a feeling of tiredness
- increased headaches, dizziness, insomnia or restlessness

If you think you might have an infection, call your doctor right away. He or she may prescribe an antibiotic for it. If an antibiotic is prescribed, **take all the medicine as directed** so it can get rid of all the infection.

When you have COPD, it is very important for you to get a flu shot each year. You may also need a pneumonia vaccine. If you do, you should be re-vaccinated every 6 years, as a rule. Ask your doctor for more information.

When to call your doctor

You need to know the first signs of an infection or respiratory problem that call for immediate treatment. Discuss these symptoms with your doctor. He or she may want you to get in touch at once when one or more of these occur:

- more shortness of breath, trouble breathing or wheezing than usual
- more coughing (more often, more severe or both)
- increase or decrease in mucus production
- change in color of mucus (to yellow, gray, green or bloody)
- swelling in ankles, legs or around eyes
- sudden weight gain (3 or more pounds overnight)
- heart palpitations or faster pulse than usual
- unusual dizziness, sleepiness, headaches, vision problems, irritability, trouble thinking
- loss of appetite (more than usual)
- dehydration (shown by darker urine and dry skin)
- fever over 101°F (38°C)
- early morning headaches not relieved by mild headache medicines (especially if you are on oxygen while sleeping)

Doctor's number: Dr. Walker 8709354150 Dr majewski 8709343530

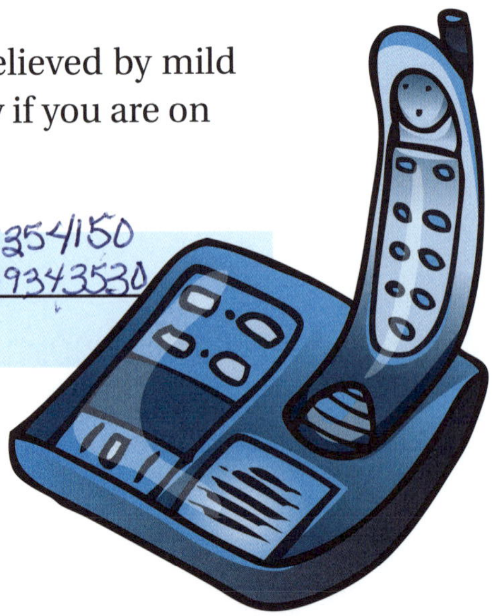

Saving energy

When you have COPD, it is important for you to learn how to avoid fatigue. You want to find the easiest ways to do your work and find a good balance between work and rest. Finding ways to conserve your energy will help you cope with your lung condition on a daily basis. It's OK to:

- change the way you do a task
- work at your own pace with breaks between tasks
- quit when you are tired
- be less than perfect

Here are some tips to help you conserve energy so you can do the things you need and want to do:

- Always walk and move slowly. DON'T RUSH.
- Use deep breathing techniques and pursed lip breathing. Exhale during the hard part of tasks.
- Combine tasks when possible.
- Plan ahead—arrange your work area so that all needed items are within easy reach.
- Don't try to do everything at once. Spread your tasks out over the entire day or week.

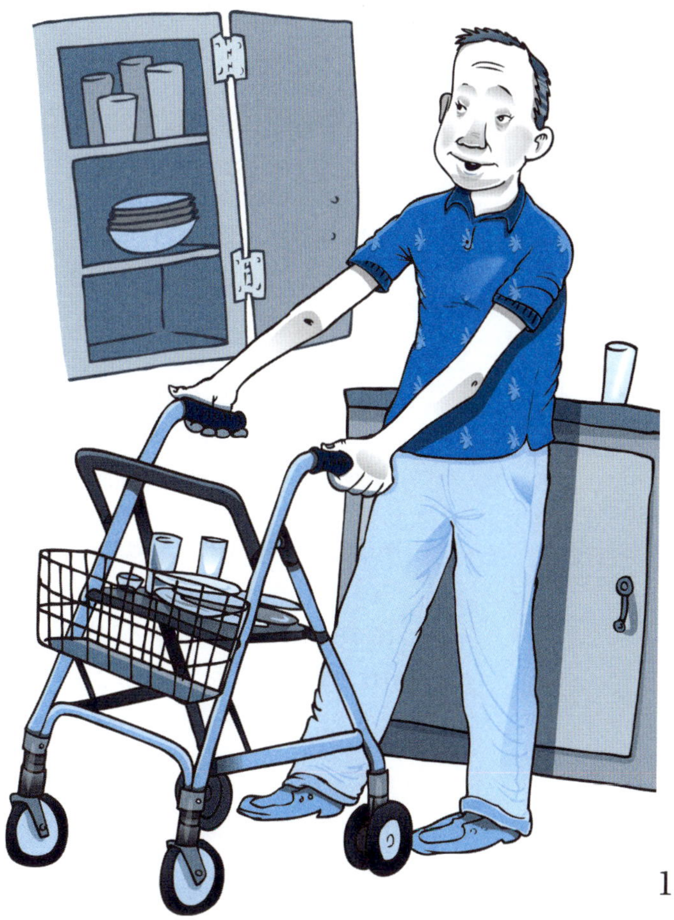

- Sit for as many activities as possible, leaning on your arms. Use a kitchen stool when working at the counter or sink.
- Determine your "best breathing" time of day for activities. Do difficult tasks during this time. If mornings are hard, shower in the evening and prepare for breakfast before bed.
- Use a terry cloth robe after your shower instead of drying yourself. Use a shower chair with a hand-held shower. Leave the bathroom door open and use the ventilation fan.
- When cooking, prepare extra food for freezing and easy reheating later.
- If possible, use a cart for carrying several items so only one trip is needed.
- Decide which tasks have to be done to make your home comfortable.
- When making the bed, make one side, sit and rest as needed, then move to the other side.
- When getting ready to leave the house, dress with enough time left to rest or use your inhaler if needed before you leave.
- When unloading the dishwasher, move the dishes from the dishwasher to the counter first. Then move the dishes from the counter to the cabinets.
- Avoid bending and lifting.

Remember, by planning ahead and working at your own pace, anything is possible!

Exercise

When you have COPD, a regular exercise program can provide many benefits. By doing aerobic and breathing exercises, you can help your body work better.

Aerobic exercise

Walking is the best aerobic exercise for you to do. You must be able to walk comfortably in order to take care of yourself and reach your goal of enjoying life to the fullest with your family and friends.

No matter how severe your lung disease is, you will most likely be able to walk farther than you think. By using your pursed lip breathing and going at a slower pace, you will find that each day you can go further.

When you begin, start slowly. If you can only go 10 steps, that's OK. If you begin to feel your chest tighten or you feel short of breath, sit down or lean against a wall or counter. Use your pursed lip breathing to regain control of your breathing. Then you can walk back to where you started.

If you have a wheelchair, you may find it helpful to walk behind it holding the handles. You can put your oxygen container in the seat of the chair. You can sit and rest if you need to. It may help to use other things (such as a grocery cart) to support you when you walk. This type of support raises your shoulders, which makes it easier to breathe.

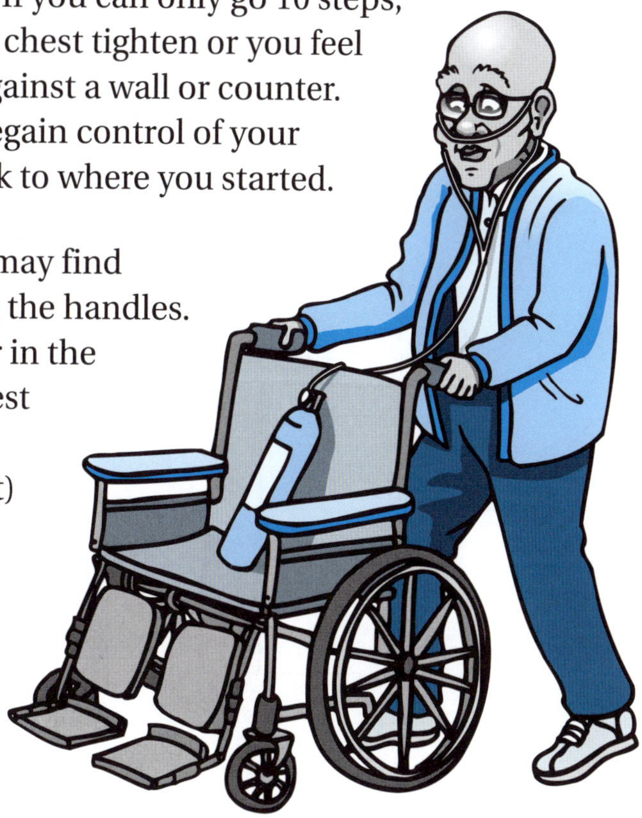

Outside factors like cold, heat, humidity, wind and pollution affect your ability to walk outside. Some days are just not good breathing days. On these days, take short walks around your house or in a store that has shopping carts. Use handicapped parking so you are close to the door.

Walking can make you stronger, improve your sense of well-being and reduce shortness of breath. It may be helpful to keep a daily record of your walking distance. Use this chart to get started.

Date	Distance walked	How you felt

If you use oxygen, ask your doctor how much to use when working on your walking program. If exercise makes you cough or wheeze, use your bronchodilator 15–30 minutes before you begin.

Breathing exercises

Do some exercise each day. Start out by building strength in your breathing muscles. This means your diaphragm and stomach muscles.

With COPD, your diaphragm flattens out. It doesn't do its normal share of the work of breathing. The work must be done by the muscles around your rib cage and in your neck and shoulders. To strengthen your diaphragm, practice **diaphragmatic breathing** along with pursed lip breathing. You might also include in your daily routine other exercises which strengthen the diaphragm and stomach muscles.

Do these exercises slowly. **Don't strain.** By learning diaphragmatic and pursed lip breathing and doing other exercises to make your body strong, you will breathe better and feel better. **Think of yourself as an active person who knows how to exercise for easy breathing.** Ask your doctor or respiratory therapist which exercises are best for you.

You can also ask about pulmonary rehabilitation (rehab) programs in your area. These programs are led by health professionals who can help you learn how to do these exercises the right way and feel better.

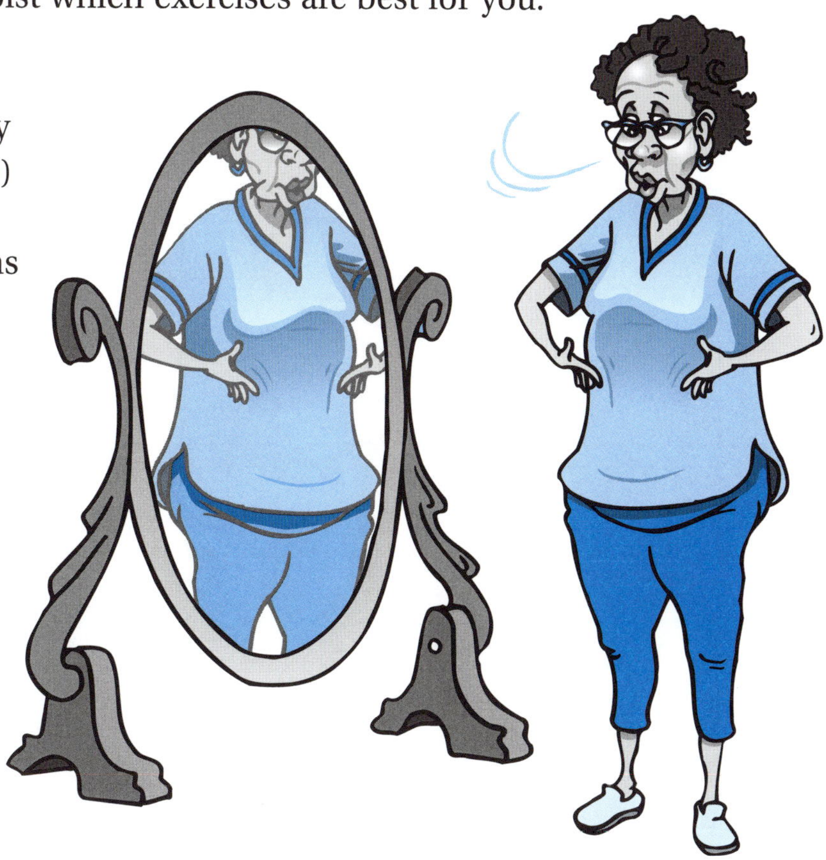

Diaphragmatic breathing

You can tell how your diaphragm works by:

- feeling it move on the front of your abdomen
- feeling it move on the sides of your abdomen

Exercise 1: Front

1. **Sit comfortably** with good posture or **lie on your back** with your head and knees supported by pillows.
2. Place one hand on your chest to check for movement of the rib cage muscles.
3. Place the other hand in the middle of your stomach to feel movement of the diaphragm.
4. Pull your stomach muscles **in as you exhale** slowly through pursed lips.
5. Inhale through your nose, feeling your stomach relax and **move out to the front.**
6. Rest after 3 or 4 breaths.

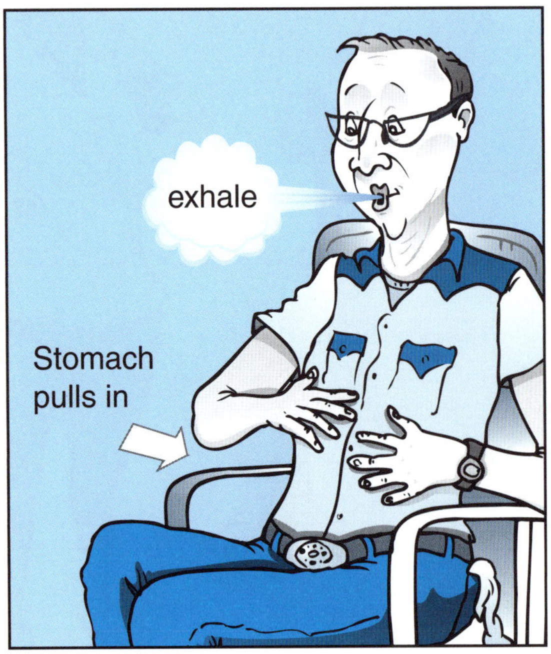

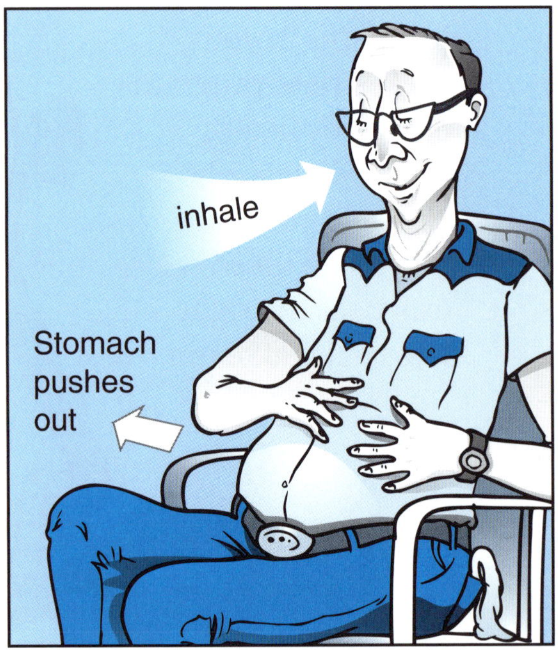

Exercise 2: Side

1. Sit or stand comfortably with good posture.
2. Place your hands on your sides over your lower ribs.
3. Feel your **lower ribs move down as you exhale** slowly through pursed lips.
4. **Inhale** slowly through your nose, feeling your **lower ribs expand.**
5. Rest after 3 or 4 breaths.

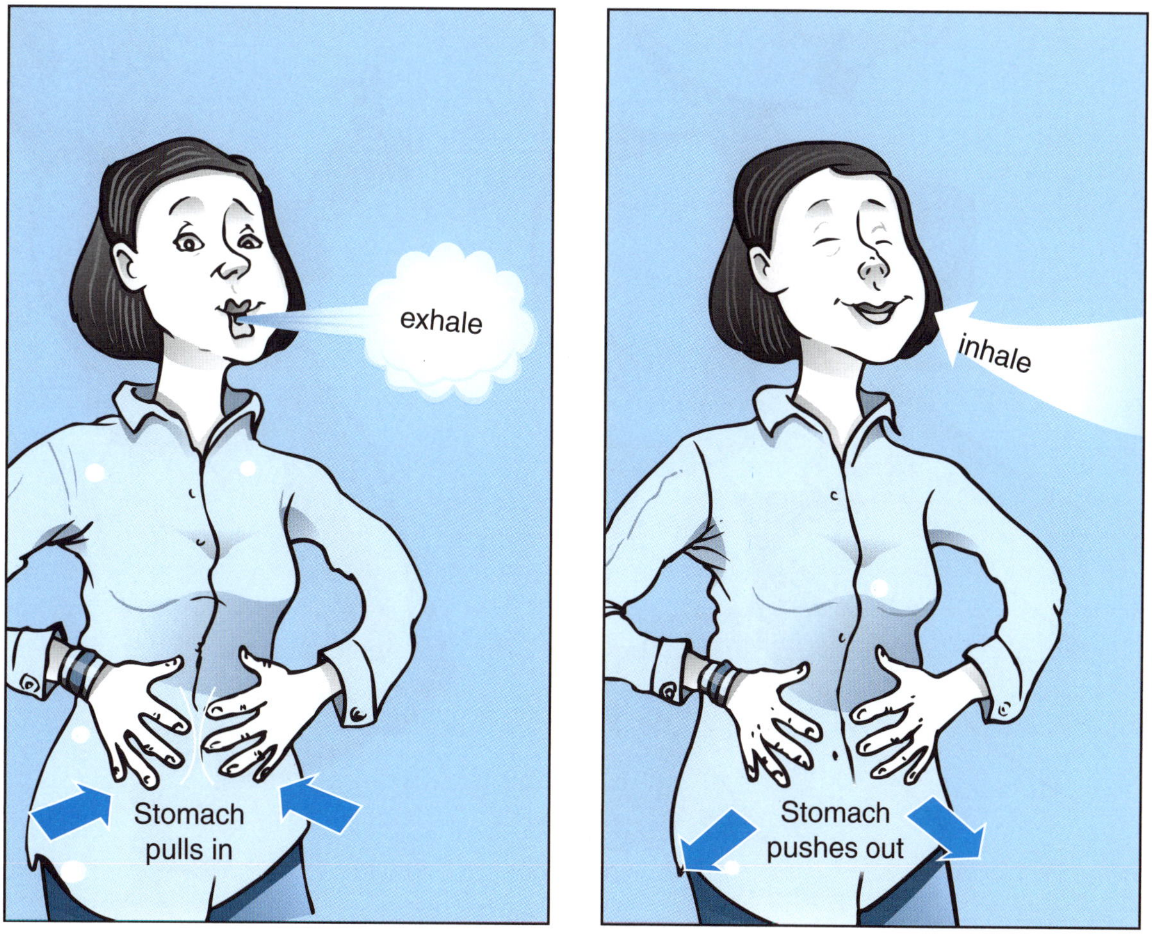

To begin with, practice both exercises 2 or 3 times a day. When you learn to do these 2 exercises well, you can make diaphragmatic breathing your normal way of breathing.

Whenever you exercise or work around the house, use diaphragmatic and pursed lip breathing. **Exhale while you do the "work" part of an exercise.** For example, exhale during a sit-up; inhale while lying back down. If you are climbing stairs, exhale as you step up and pause to inhale.

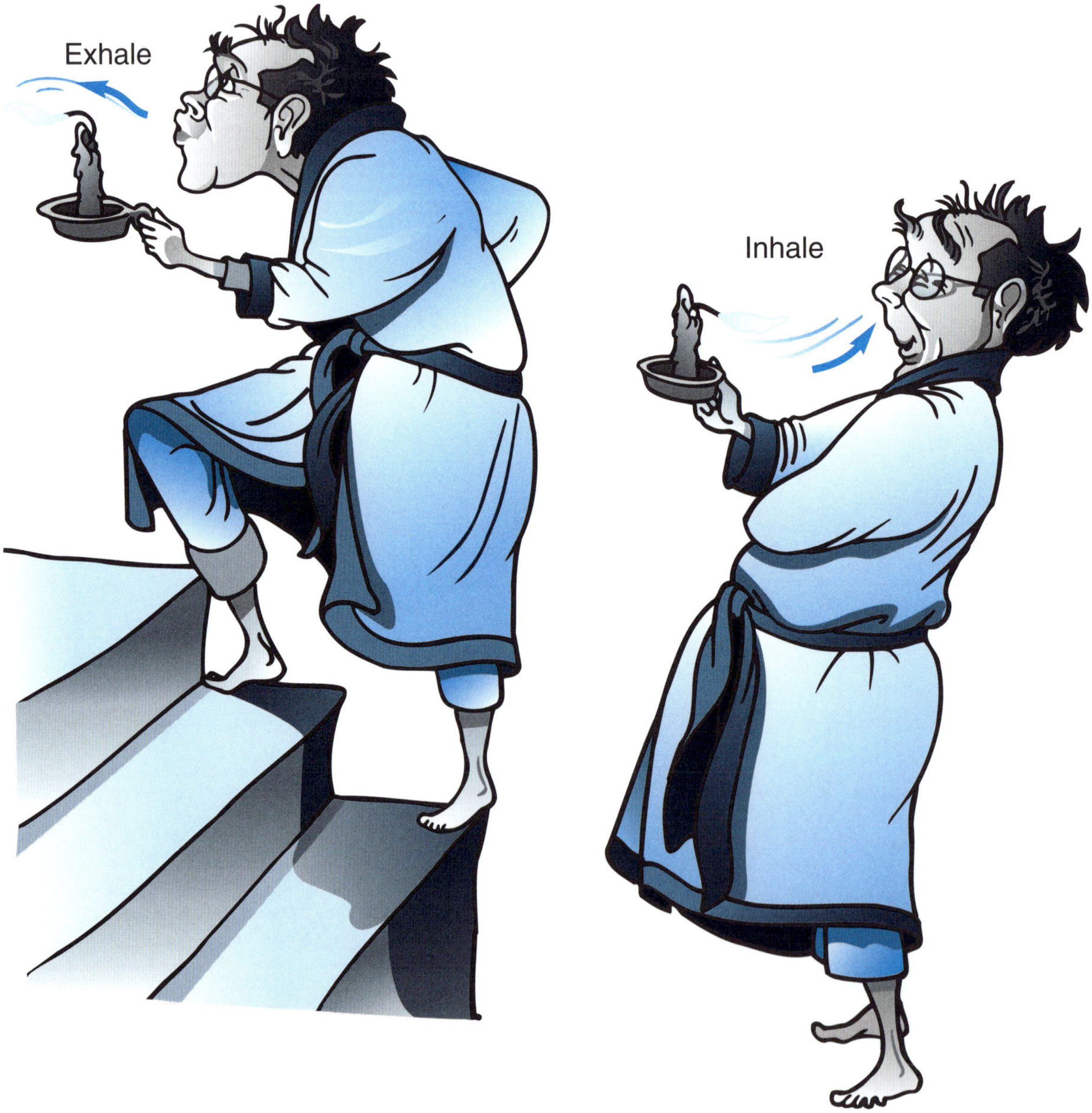

Breathing retraining exercises

These exercises help you breathe better by building strength in your stomach muscles. Practice them each day. Do not do them when you feel sick or short of breath. Ask your doctor if these are OK for you.

Butterfly

1. Sit up straight in a chair with your arms at your sides and your feet flat on the floor. Keep your back straight against the chair back.
2. Place your hands behind your head and raise Your elbows to be even with your shoulders. Breathe in slowly through your nose.
3. As you breathe out slowly through pursed lips, slowly bend over toward your knees, bringing your elbows in towards your face. Bend over only as far as is comfortable.
4. Inhale as you slowly return to a sitting position.
5. Rest.

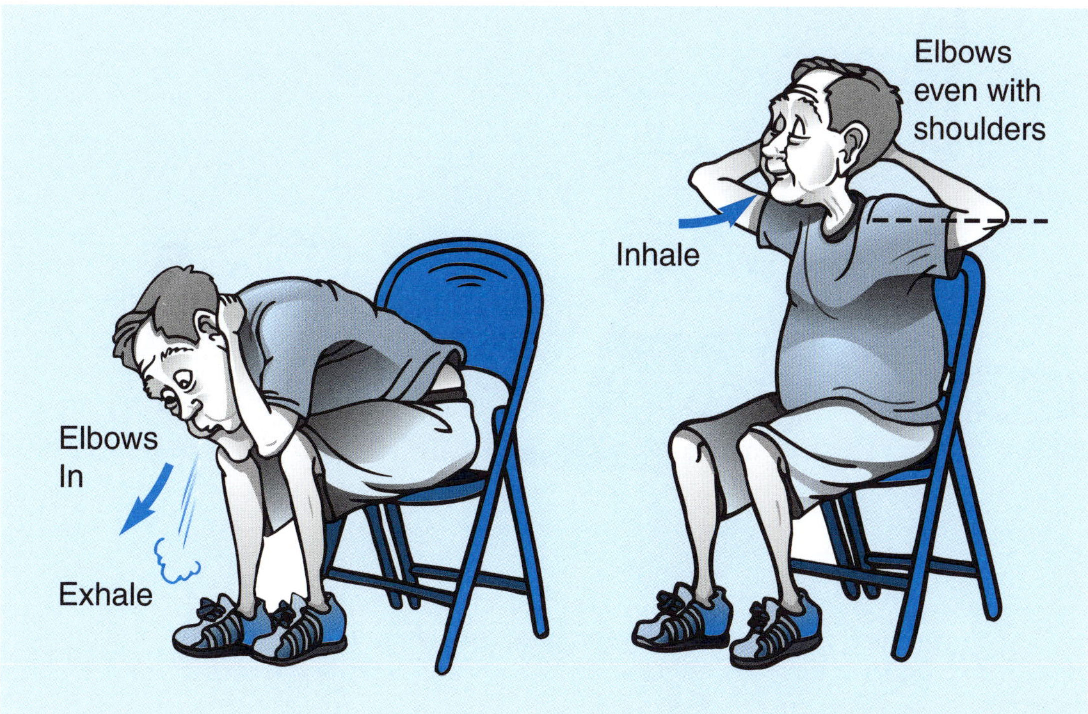

Knee to chest

1. Lie **flat on your back*** on the floor with your knees bent and your feet flat on the floor.

2. Inhale slowly through your nose.

3. As you slowly exhale through pursed lips, bring your left knee to your chest.

4. Use your hands to pull your knee tightly towards your chest.

5. As you inhale through your nose, slowly lower your left foot to the floor.

6. Rest.

7. Repeat with your right leg.

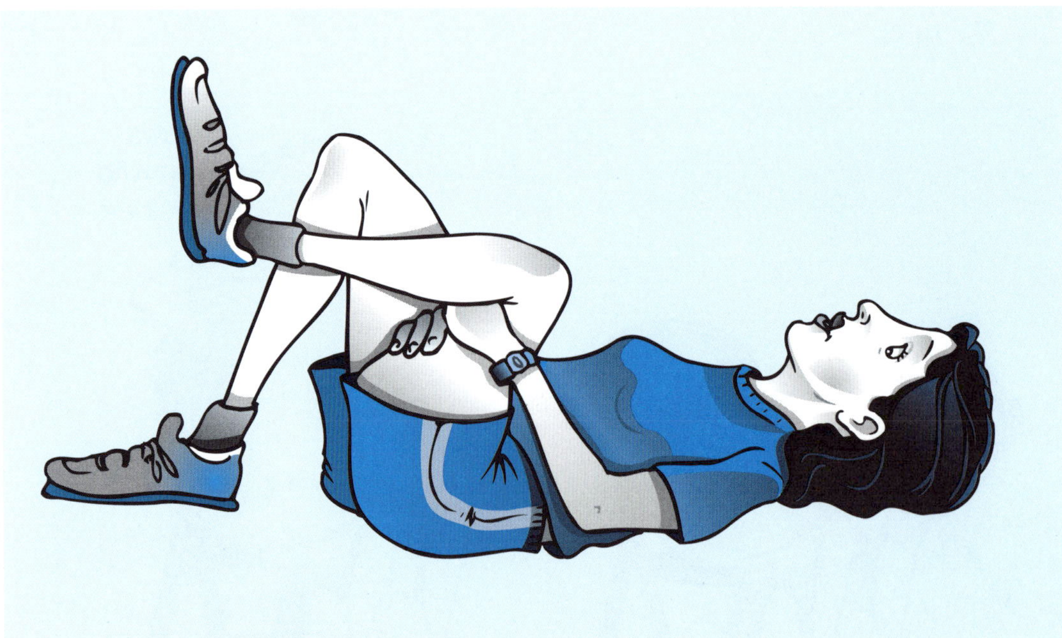

**If you can't lie flat, support your head and chest with pillows.*

Chapter 2

Normal Lungs and Lung Diseases

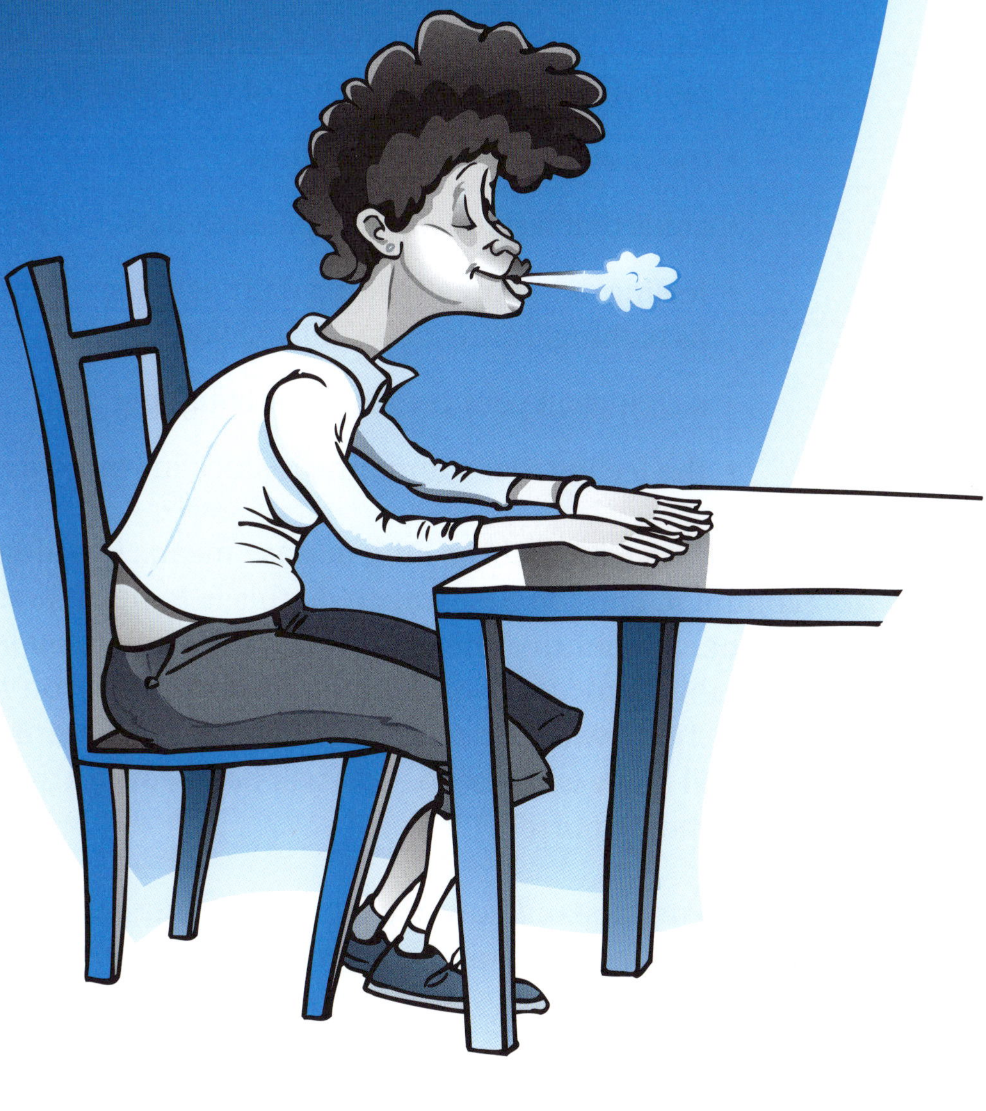

A word about COPD

COPD stands for chronic obstructive pulmonary disease. *Chronic* means long-term. *Obstructive* refers to blockage in the airways of the lung. *Pulmonary* refers to the lungs.

The most common obstructive lung diseases are chronic bronchitis, emphysema, asthma, bronchiectasis and cystic fibrosis (CF). With COPD, you may have one or more of these symptoms:

- shortness of breath
- a chronic cough or heavy sputum (phlegm or mucus)
- wheezing (a high-pitched whistling sound caused by air trying to move in and out of your airways)
- too much mucus in your lungs
- colds that last for weeks instead of days
- feeling out of breath doing daily activities (such as bathing, eating or walking to your car)
- a change in your breathing or coughing
- the feeling that something is stuck in your chest

Living with chronic lung disease means learning to control it, and the best way to do this is to be an active partner in your treatment. Practice daily what you learn from this book. Ask your doctor any questions you may have. Then, when breathing problems or infections occur, you will know what to do. You will be in control and feel good about yourself.

To understand how to deal with lung disease, it may first be helpful to understand how normal lungs work.

Normal lungs and normal breathing

Each time you **breathe in** (inspiration), your body gets the **oxygen** it needs to live. Each time you **breathe out** (expiration), your body gets rid of **carbon dioxide** which it produces as waste. Your lungs remove carbon dioxide from the blood so you can exhale it.

If your air supply were cut off for about 5 minutes, your body would run out of the oxygen it needs. And if you couldn't exhale the carbon dioxide your body makes, the buildup in your blood would soon cause headaches, fatigue (tiredness) and drowsiness.

Most of the work to get air in and out of your lungs is done by your **diaphragm.** This is a sheet of muscle that separates your chest from your stomach cavity **(abdomen).** Your lungs are sealed in an airtight cavity. When your diaphragm moves down, this airtight cavity expands. This creates a vacuum which sucks air into your lungs. When your diaphragm relaxes, it lets air flow back out of your lungs.

Air enters your body through your mouth or nose. Your mouth and nose clean the air and bring it to the right moisture and body temperature. The air then enters your windpipe **(trachea)** and flows through large air tubes **(bronchi)** to your lungs. The right lung has 3 parts, or **lobes,** and the left lung has 2.

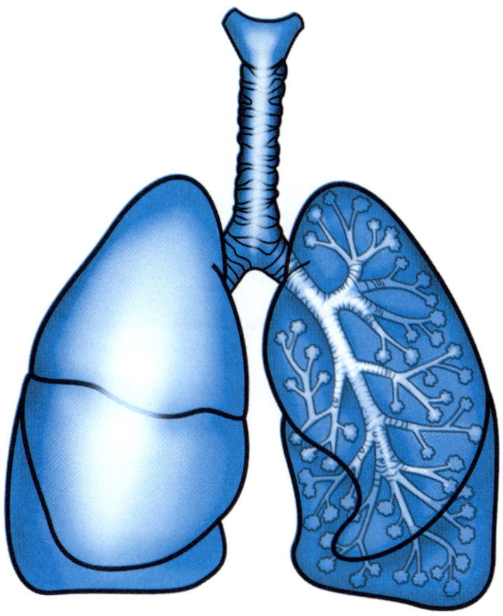

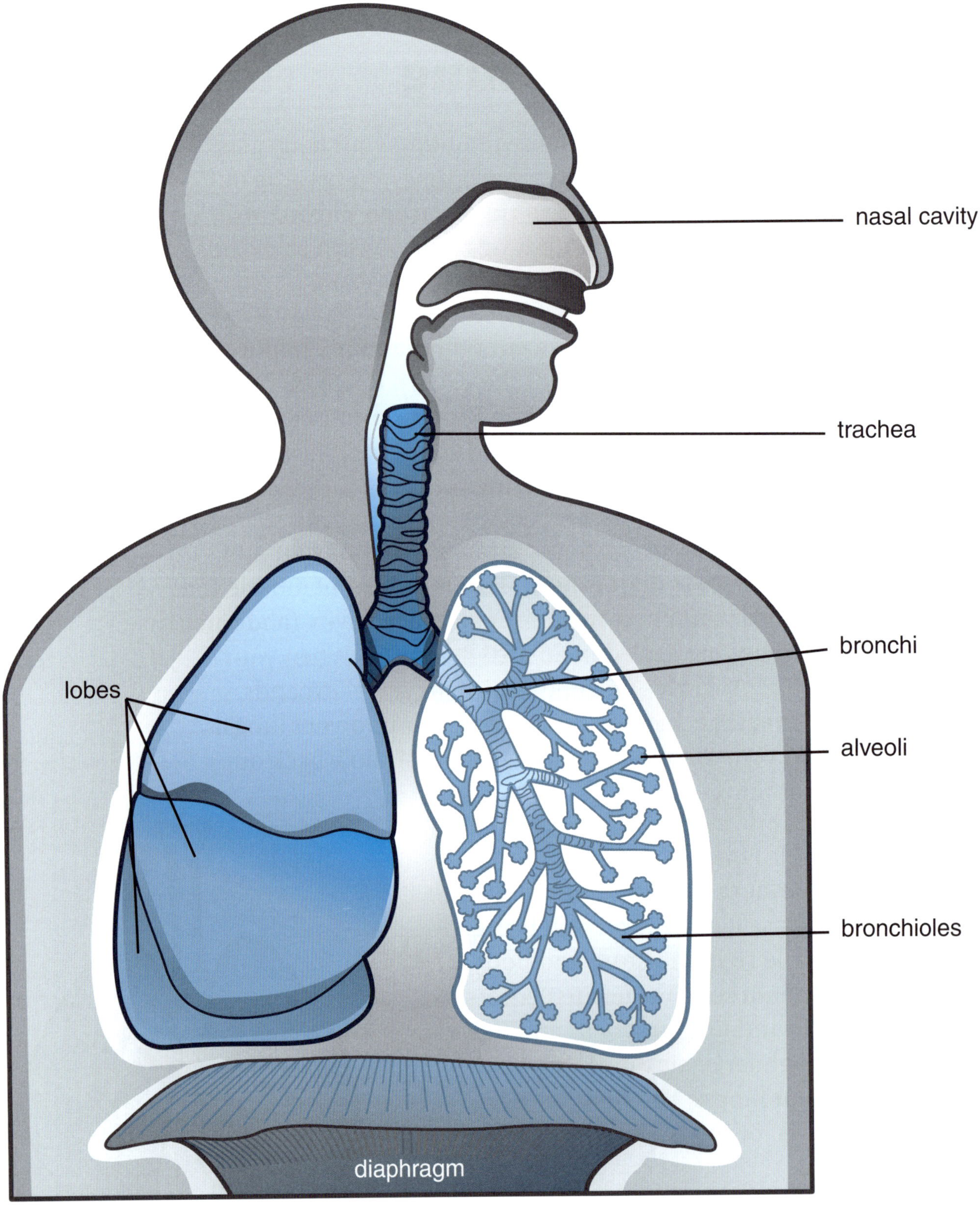
nasal cavity
trachea
bronchi
lobes
alveoli
bronchioles
diaphragm

The bronchi supply all parts of your lungs with air by splitting again and again into smaller bronchi which run through all 5 lobes of your lungs. Your bronchi divide into even smaller air tubes **(bronchioles)** and end finally in 300 million tiny, elastic air sacs **(alveoli).**

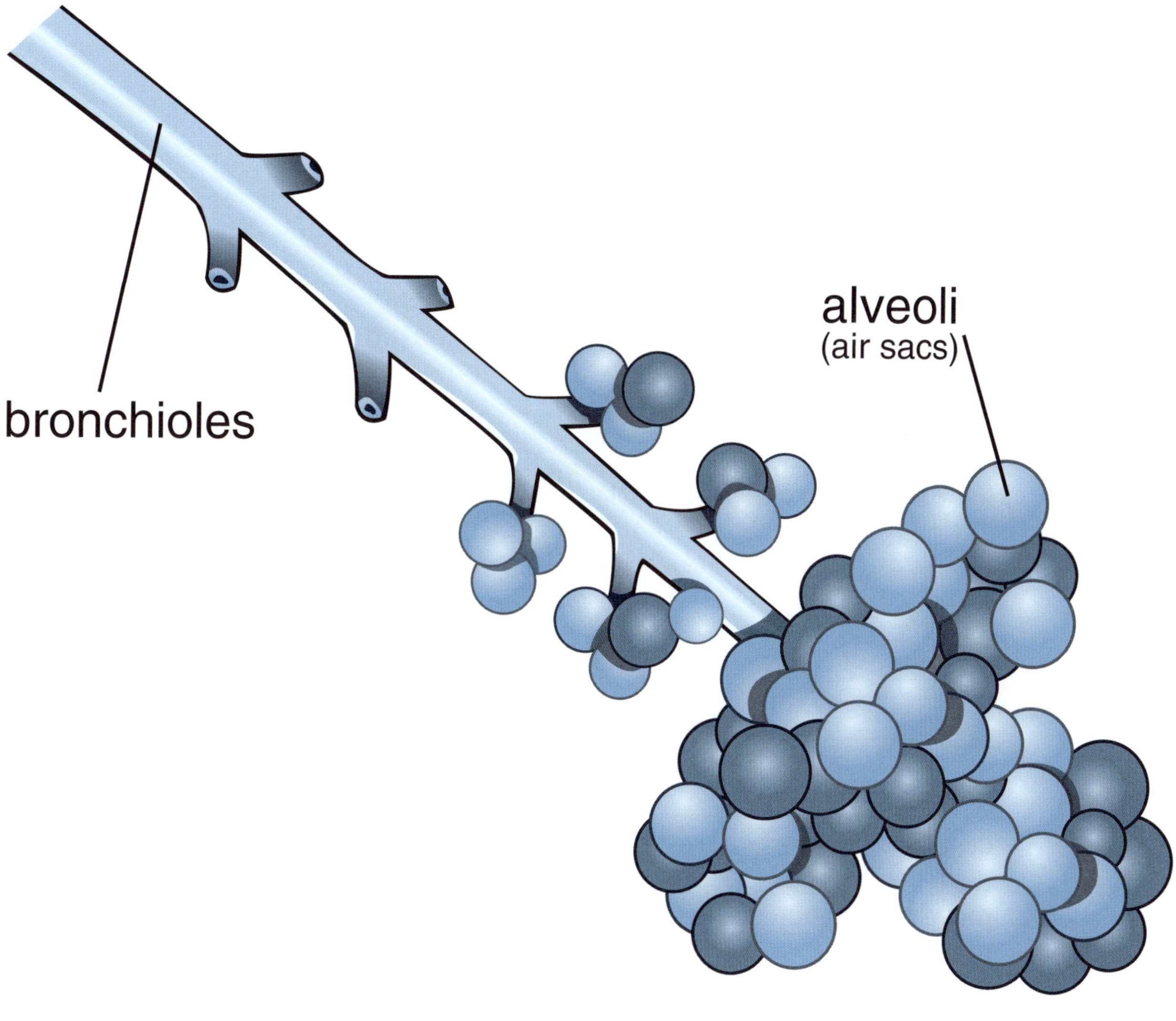

If the air which enters your lungs contains gases or dirt particles, the airways in your lungs have a system to clean it. All breathing tubes are lined with mucus and cells which have tiny hairs **(cilia).** Other cells in your airways make mucus which lies on top of the cilia. You have millions of cilia, all sweeping mucus toward your throat. Inhaled dirt particles are trapped on the mucus and are pushed up the windpipe. There you swallow it or cough it out. So, by the time air reaches your alveoli, it is clean. The oxygen is ready to be picked up by your blood and carried to all parts of your body.

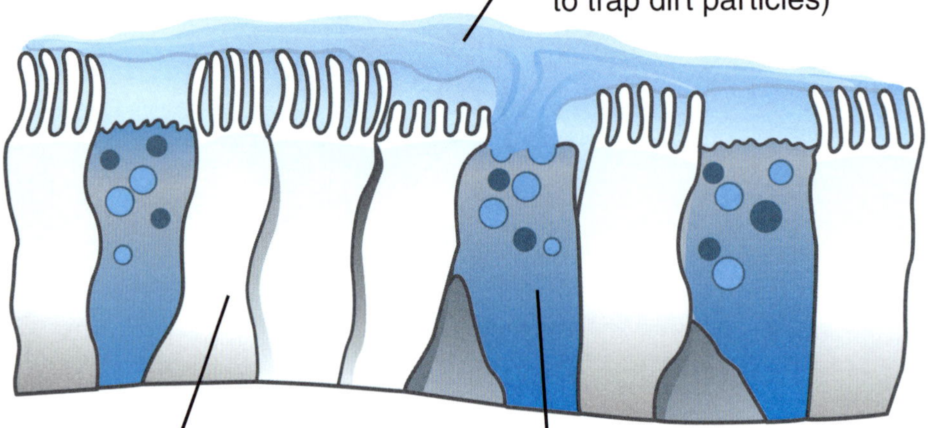

The walls of your alveoli are about as thick as a soap bubble just before it bursts. Running through these walls are tiny blood tubes **(capillaries).** Your lungs have about 3 billion capillaries. Oxygen easily passes into these tiny blood tubes from your air sacs. All carbon dioxide crosses into the air sacs where it is left to be exhaled.

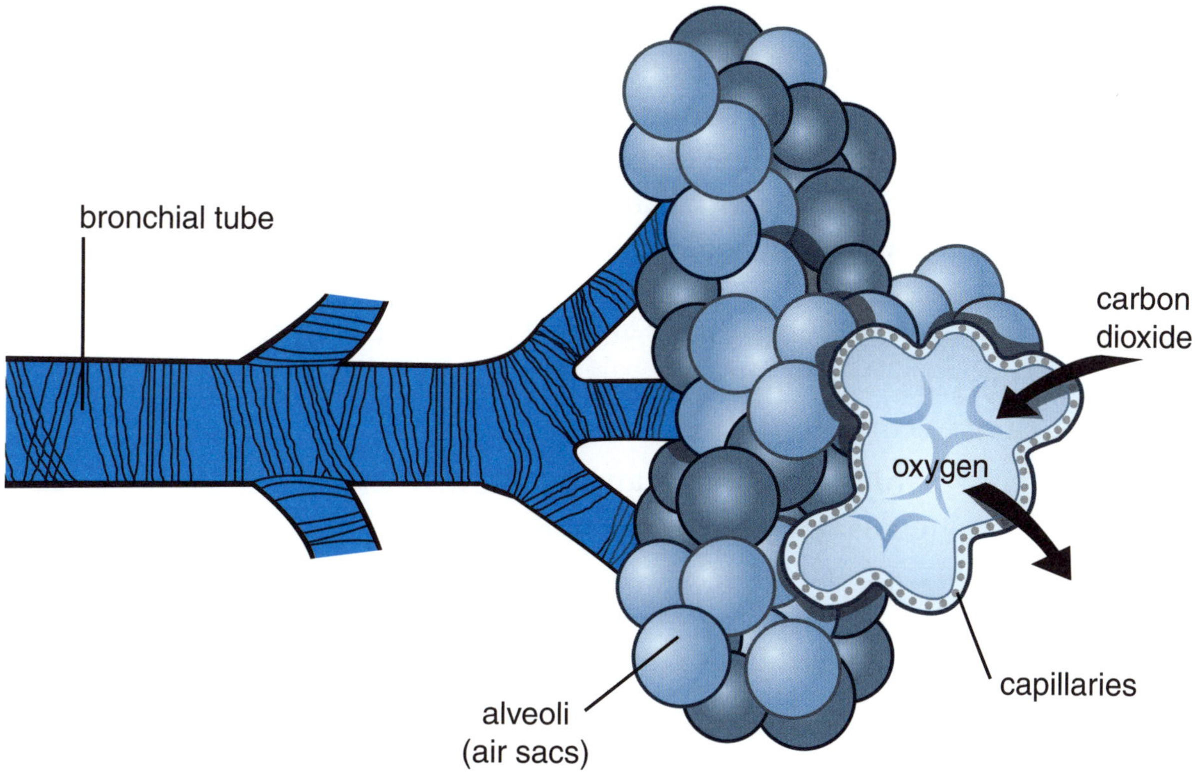

Now that you understand how normal lungs work, let's look at the five most common diseases of the lungs.

Ask your doctor to check which of these you have.

Chronic bronchitis

Chronic bronchitis is an **inflammation of the lining of your bronchial tubes.** They become inflamed (red and swollen) and then make too much mucus. This can be brought on by:

- cigarette smoke
- air pollution
- allergens

Any of these may irritate (bother) the lining of your bronchial tubes. It becomes harder to breathe, and the extra mucus causes chronic coughing and wheezing. Some air tubes may even be blocked by excess mucus. When this happens, you are more likely to have lung infections. These can do lasting damage to your lungs.

Antibiotics can cure bacterial infections, but they can't cure chronic bronchitis itself. The best way to stop the progress of chronic bronchitis is to:

- **avoid the irritant causing the disease (especially cigarette smoke)**
- drink a lot of fluids, especially water
- keep your lungs cleared of mucus
- take the medicines prescribed for you

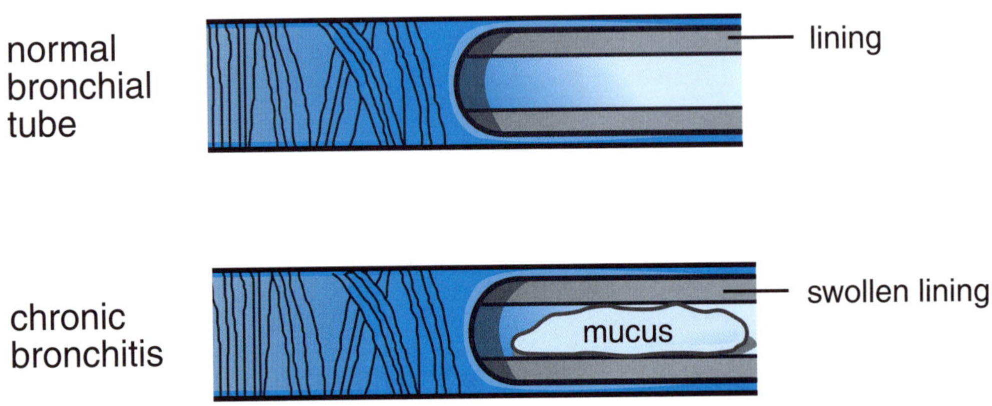

Emphysema

Emphysema is a disease which **destroys your air sacs.** It also causes airway blockage. Most emphysema is caused by cigarette smoke. The air sacs, blood vessels and support tissue are destroyed. Many of the small air tubes collapse. With emphysema:

- The transfer of oxygen and carbon dioxide does not occur as it should.
- Extra pressure is needed to exhale; some small and even some large airways (bronchial tubes) may collapse, so your body has to work harder to get air out.
- More mucus may be trapped in your lungs, making them prone to infection.
- You suffer from shortness of breath and coughing.
- Over time, your lungs and even your heart may become enlarged.
- Your chest becomes rounded (barrel-shaped).

Emphysema has no cure. But medications and breathing exercises help. **Not smoking** and avoiding other irritants will help slow the progress of the disease.

Most people with COPD have both emphysema and bronchitis.

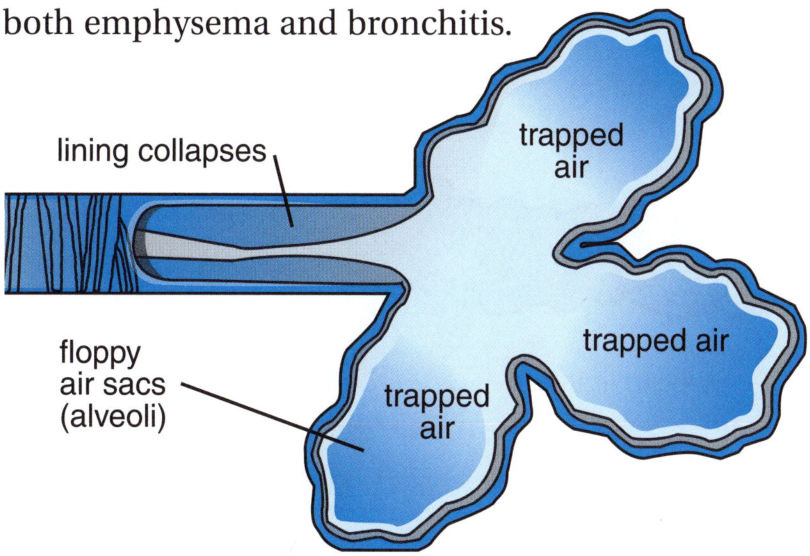

Asthma

If you have asthma, your **airways** become tighter, **inflamed and swollen.** They also make **extra mucus.** The muscles in the walls of these airways also go into **spasm** and clamp down on the airways. These changes make it hard for air to flow in and out of your lungs. These are called **asthma flare-ups.**

During an asthma flare-up (attack or episode), you may:

- cough
- be short of breath
- have chest tightness
- wheeze (a high-pitched whistling sound made by air trying to move in and out of your airways)

Things that cause asthma flare-ups are called triggers. There are many types, and they vary from person to person. Colds and flus, smoke, dust mites, exercise and things you are allergic to are some of the more common triggers. The best way to prevent an asthma flare-up is to avoid your triggers.

If you have asthma or think you have asthma, ask your doctor for more information about how to treat it.

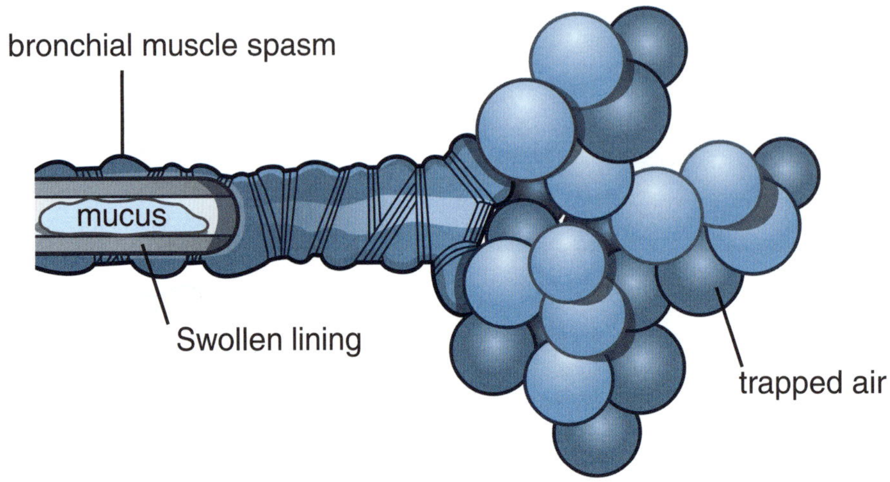

Bronchiectasis

Bronchiectasis can be caused by:

- a serious lung infection, often in early childhood
- abnormal lung development before birth or during childhood

It is common in people who have cystic fibrosis. In bronchiectasis, **scar tissue** which **makes too much mucus** replaces the walls of your airways. The airways deep in your lungs become widened sacs where mucus can pool. Your mucus membrane and bronchial muscles are not able to push this pooled mucus up to your throat to be expelled (spit out or swallowed). So you may cough, wheeze and suffer from shortness of breath and excess mucus. You may also have persistent infection from the mucus.

Treatment includes water drinking, antibiotics, pursed lip breathing and use of bronchodilators.

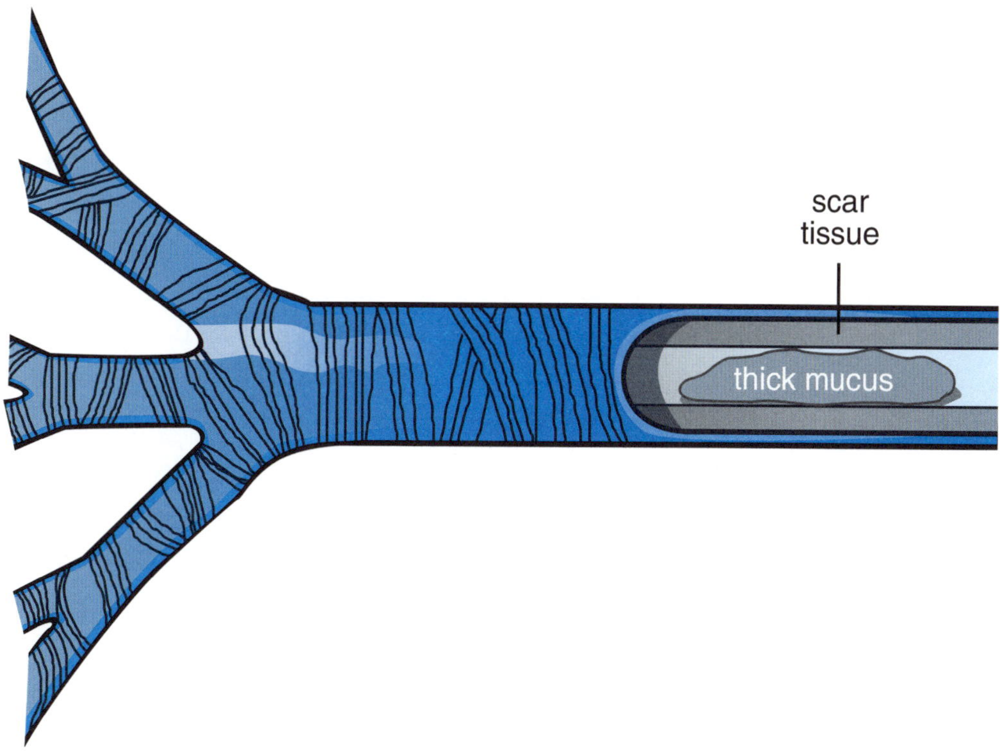

Cystic fibrosis

Cystic fibrosis (CF) affects the lungs and the digestive system. People with CF are born with it, though it sometimes does not show up until later. They inherit the disease in the genes they get from their parents.

In the lungs of a person with CF, thick, sticky mucus blocks the airways. This makes breathing harder and causes coughing and wheezing. Because of these blockages, the lungs become infected easily and often. This leads to lasting damage of the alveoli, bronchioles and bronchi.

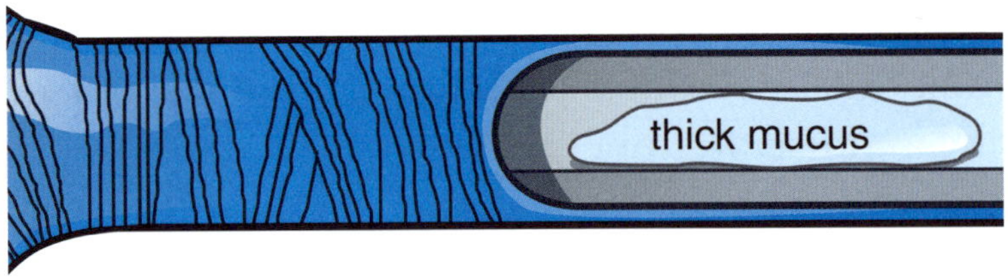

Treatment for the respiratory problems caused by CF includes using antibiotics to keep the lungs as clear of infection as possible. You can help prevent problems by doing breathing exercises and postural drainage, drinking a lot of fluids, especially water, and using aerosol therapy and bronchodilators.

CF has no cure, but with early diagnosis and use of antibiotics for lung infections, it can be managed. Continuing advances in diagnosis and treatment offer longer, better quality lives for people with CF.

Chapter 3

Managing COPD

CAUTION:

Do not take any of the drugs described in this section unless prescribed by your doctor.

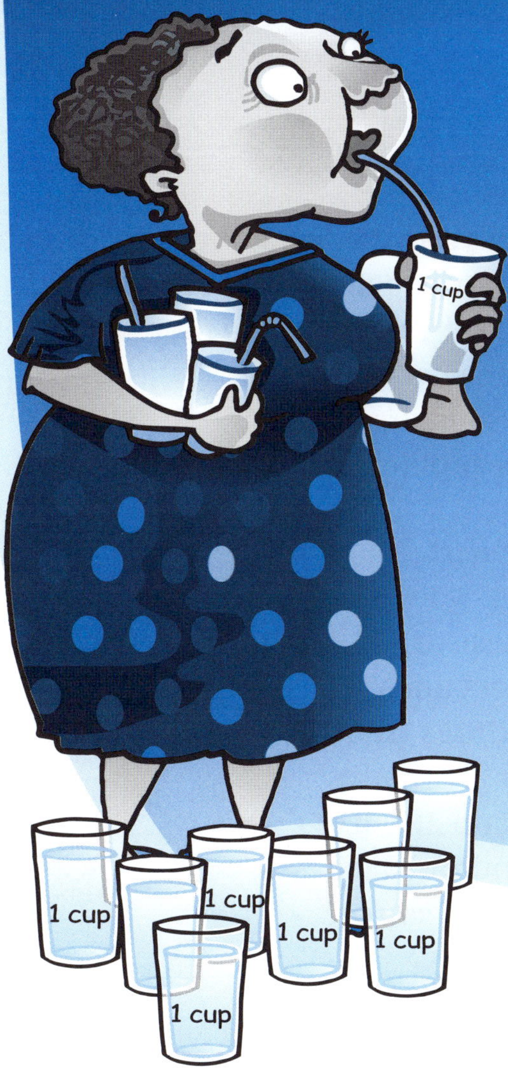

Management

Managing COPD is the key to keeping your lungs and airways expanded and clear of blockage. Ask your doctor about the treatments that are right for you (see page 79).

Medications

The following pages cover most of the drugs prescribed for lung disease. These include:

- bronchodilators
- anti-inflammatory medicines
- antibiotics
- cough medicines

Learn which drugs you take, what they are for and their side effects. Tell your doctor if you feel these side effects at any time. Also, if you are taking more than one drug, your pharmacist can keep a list of them for you. Sometimes drugs may interact and cause problems.

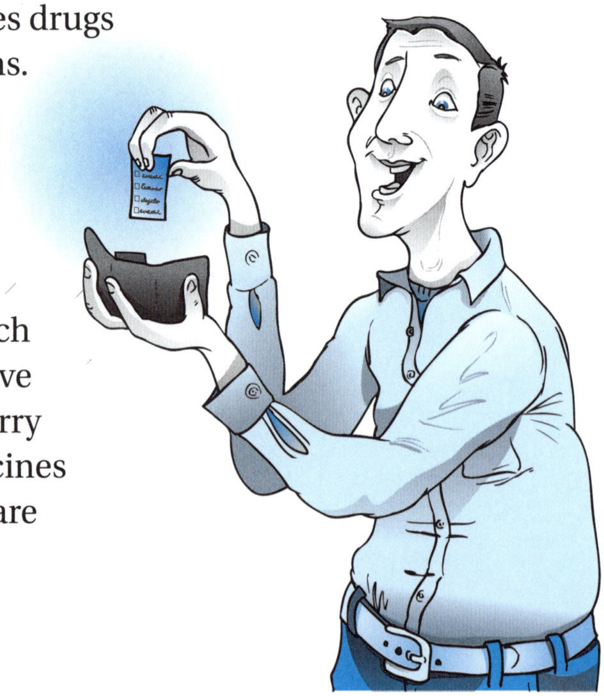

Bring a medicine chart that lists all of the drugs you are taking. Include those drugs ordered by other doctors and any over-the-counter drugs (such as eye drops, herbal or alternative supplements and vitamins). Carry an up-to-date list of your medicines in your purse or wallet. If you are having trouble breathing or can't speak, this list can be very helpful to the doctor treating you.

Bronchodilators

These drugs relax the muscles around the bronchial tubes. The tubes open up, and you breathe easier. These drugs can be taken by pills, shots, liquids or aerosol sprays.

Use bronchodilators only as your doctor tells you. Take the amount prescribed at the times he or she tells you. Use this inhaler first if you are also scheduled to use a steroid inhaler. If this medicine upsets your stomach, take it with food. Call your doctor if any of these side effects occur:

- ✗ irregular heartbeat
- ✗ nervousness, restlessness
- ✗ trembling
- ✗ bad taste in mouth
- ✗ headache
- ✗ trouble sleeping
- ✗ nausea/vomiting or stomach pain
- ✗ urinating more often

Xanthines (Theophylline)

(examples include Theo-Dur®, Uni-dur®, Uniphyl® and Theo-24®)

- Take doses at evenly divided times during the day (example: twice a day—take every 12 hours).
- Do not take on an empty stomach.
- If your doctor tells you to, avoid or limit the amounts of coffee, tea or sodas with caffeine in them.
- Do not chew tablets.
- Do not take more medicine than you're told to.
- Cigarette smoke affects theophylline levels. Let your doctor know if you or someone in your home smokes or recently stopped.
- Let your doctor know if you are placed on any new medicine (especially antibiotics, ulcer or seizure medicine).

❑ *Beta agonists (inhalers)*

There are two types of Beta agonist inhalers:

– **Quick Acting**

- Albuterol (Ventolin®, Proventil®)
- Pirbuterol (Maxair Autohaler®)

Quick acting inhalers are known as rescue breathers and are used to relieve shortness of breath. They act within 5-15 minutes to relieve your stress.

– **Long Acting**

- Serevent®
- Foradil Aerolizer®

Long acting inhalers will not relieve your shortness of breath right away. But the dose will last for 12 hours to help you breathe better 24 hours a day.

Other things to know

- Know how to use the inhaler properly (see page 51).
- A spacer may be prescribed.
- Use only the amount your doctor tells you and only as often as directed.
- If you are using more than one puff for your dose, wait a few minutes between puffs. The first puff opens your airways so the second puff can get deeper.
- Store the inhaler away from heat and direct sunlight.

❑ *Beta agonists (pill or liquid)*

(examples include Volmax®, Proventil® and Repetabs®)

- Take only the dose your doctor prescribes.
- Do not take this drug more often than directed.

❑ *Anticholinergics (inhalers)*

(examples include Atrovent® and Spiriva®)

This type of drug is not used for quick-relief. It takes effect more slowly than other kinds of bronchodilators.

– **Atrovent®**

This is inhaled using a metered dose inhaler (MDI [see page 51]) or using a nebulizer (see page 54). Take doses at evenly spaced times per day (example: 3 times a day—take every 8 hours).

Before you take Atrovent®, **let your doctor know if you have glaucoma (an eye disease) or difficulty urinating**. This drug makes these problems worse.

– **Spiriva®**

This is inhaled using a dry powered inhaler (DPI). The DPI it uses is a HandiHaler® (see page 53) that uses capsules packaged in a blister card. Take one dose each day.

If you are allergic to **lactose, atropine or any drugs like it, you should not take this drug.**

Combination inhalers

❑ – **Combivent®**

This is an inhaler that contains two different bronchodilators:

- Albuterol (a beta agonist)
- Atrovent (an anticholinergic)

With the puffs you take, you get both medications but only have to use one inhaler. The usual dose is 2-3 puffs every 4-6 hours, but you may only have to use this when you need it. Be sure to follow the instructions. The inhaler is your **rescue inhaler. If you are prescribed this, never leave home without it!**

❑ *Combination inhalers* (continued)

– **Advair®**

This is a combination of two different medications also:

- Flovent® (an inhaled steroid and anti-inflammatory)
- Serevent® (a long acting bronchodilator)

These can be very helpful in controlling your symptoms. Advair is inhaled using a Diskus® inhaler (see page 52). This medicine comes in 3 different strengths. Your doctor may prescribe different strengths at different times for you based on your needs.

This is **not a rescue breather**. It is long acting and will not relieve your shortness of breath quickly but should help you breathe better once you are on it on a regular basis.

Other things to know:

- Know how to use the inhaler properly (see page 52).
- The dosage is 1 puff every 12 hours or morning and night. It is important that you use it twice a day, every day.
- If using more than one puff for a dose, wait a few minutes between puffs.
- Use only the amount your doctor tells you.
- Do not store above 86° F (30° C); avoid a lot of humidity.
- It is important that you rinse out your mouth right after taking this. If you have dentures, you need to remove them and then rinse.
- It may be handy to keep it by your toothbrush and use it before you brush in the morning and again at night.
- Do not stop using it unless your doctor tells you to.
- Side effects include: coughing, dry mouth, nausea and headaches.

Anti-inflammatory medicines

Anti-inflammatory drugs decrease swelling of the airways and mucus production. They must be used regularly. They don't have immediate effects, but they help prevent shortness of breath and wheezing once they start to work.

Anti-inflammatory drugs come in various forms such as pills, shots, liquids and aerosol sprays. **Never change your dosage or stop taking anti-inflammatory drugs without your doctor's advice.**

Steroids

Oral steroids

When taken as a pill or liquid, always take with food, milk or an antacid liquid. If you have stomach pain or burning, call your doctor. Stomach problems are more likely to occur if you drink alcohol while taking steroids. Also, tell the doctor you are taking this drug:

- before having a vaccination
- before having any kind of surgery (including dental surgery)
- if you get a serious infection or injury

CAUTION:

Never stop taking steroids without your doctor's advice!

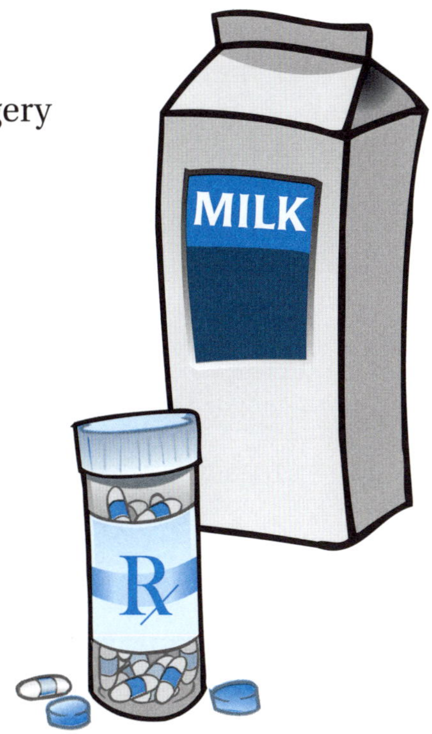

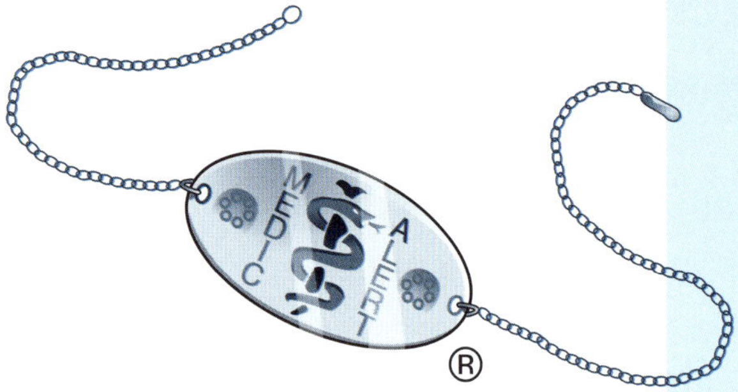

NOTE:

Wear an ID bracelet or necklace (such as Medic Alert) saying you are taking steroids long term (over 1 month).

Tell your doctor if any of these or other side effects occur:

- ❑ bloody or black stools
- ❑ back or rib pain
- ❑ decreased or blurred vision
- ❑ frequent urination or increased thirst
- ❑ acne or other skin problems
- ❑ ongoing stomach pain, burning or nausea/vomiting (your doctor may give you medicines to help with this)
- ❑ unusual tiredness or weakness
- ❑ menstrual problems
- ❑ swelling of lower legs
- ❑ changes in emotions, like depression, rapid mood changes, etc.
- ❑ weight gain (limit salt and salty foods when on oral steroids)
- ❑ easy bruising
- ❑ other: ______________________________

  ____

❑ Steroid inhalers

(examples include Vanceril®, Flovent®, Azmacort®, Aerobid®, Aerobid-M®, Pulmicort® and Advair®)

Steroid inhalers reduce inflammation, swelling and mucus. You are more likely to be given a steroid inhaler if asthma is a part of your COPD. If you are scheduled to use a bronchodilator inhaler with your steroid inhaler, use your steroid inhaler 20 minutes after your bronchodilator (see page 51). **It will take 2–4 weeks of daily use before the steroid inhaler will have its full effect.**

Store the inhaler away from heat and direct sunlight. Be sure to brush your teeth, gargle and rinse your mouth and spit after using your steroid inhaler. This may help prevent hoarseness and throat irritation. Rinsing may also help prevent thrush (Candida albicans), a fungus infection. It may be helpful to schedule your inhaler use around the times when you normally do mouth care, like first thing in the morning and right before bed.

Steroid inhalers do not cause the usual side effects of steroids taken by mouth or shot. But they might cause:

- ✘ hoarseness
- ✘ sore mouth or throat
- ✘ cough

Let your doctor know if any of these side effects occur.

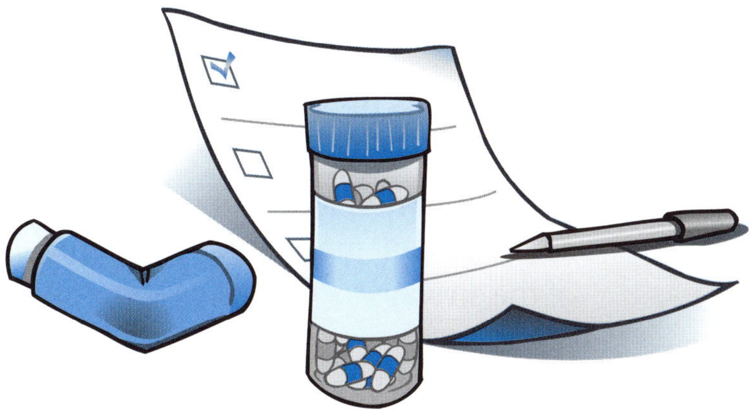

Non-steroids

- [ ] **Cromolyn sodium/Nedocromil**
(examples include Intal® and Tilade®)

Both of these drugs are inhaled. Cromolyn sodium comes in the form of **a liquid** for use in a **nebulizer** and as an **aerosol** for use in a **metered dose inhaler (MDI). Nedocromil** comes in the form of an **aerosol** for use in an **MDI.** If you are scheduled to use a bronchodilator inhaler with either of these drugs, use them 20 minutes after your bronchodilator (see page 51). **These drugs help prevent symptoms but will not provide immediate relief once symptoms start.**

Side effects are rare but may include:

- ✗ throat irritation or dryness
- ✗ bad taste in the mouth
- ✗ coughing
- ✗ wheezing
- ✗ nausea
- ✗ nasal congestion

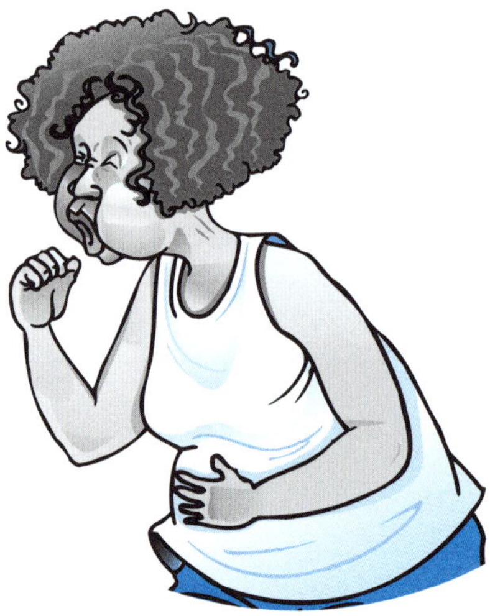

- [ ] **Leukotriene modifiers**
(examples include Accolate®, Singulair® and Zyflo®)

Leukotriene modifiers are a newer class of asthma medicines. These drugs prevent swelling of the airways.

They can be taken in pill or liquid form. They should not be taken with meals. Side effects from these medicines are rare.

Antibiotics

When you have COPD, your lungs' natural defense system does not work as well as it should. When your lungs cannot protect themselves, even a mild infection can turn out to be very serious.

If you have any signs of infection, your doctor may tell you to take antibiotics to fight bacteria and protect your lungs. There are many different kinds of antibiotics, but they must be prescribed by a doctor. They can be taken in the form of pills, capsules, liquids or shots.

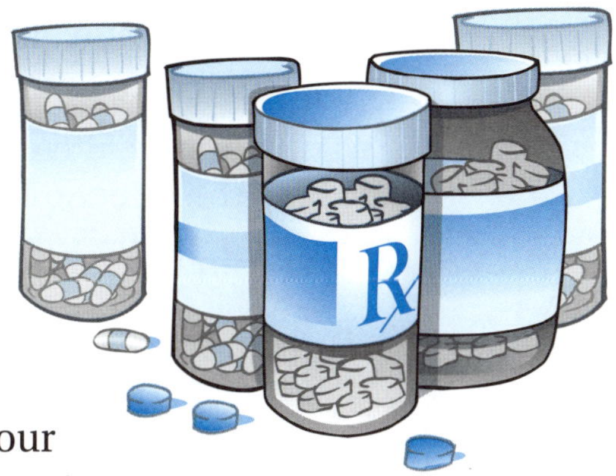

Take antibiotics just as your doctor tells you. You should also keep these things in mind:

- Take all of your antibiotic(s).
- Take your antibiotic at the same time each day.
- Don't skip any doses. If you do, your infection can last longer or get worse!
- Some of these drugs are better absorbed if you take them 30 minutes before eating and if you don't take them with milk or an antacid.
- Don't insist that your doctor prescribe an antibiotic. They only work with bacterial infections (not a cold, flu or other viral infection) and may not work if taken too often.
- Tell your doctor if you have any side effects. Side effects may include nausea, stomach cramps, diarrhea or a skin rash.
- Ask if the antibiotic may affect other medicines you take, like birth control pills.
- You may have to take it with meals.

Tell your doctor if you have any drug allergies. You should also make sure your doctor and pharmacist know all of the medicines you are taking with your antibiotic.

Take only your own antibiotic. Since each type of antibiotic only works on certain bacteria, the antibiotic someone else is taking may not work for your illness. You should also see your doctor each time you have a new infection. Don't assume that the antibiotic you used for the last infection will work for the new one.

Don't stop taking your antibiotic even if you feel better. If you don't finish the prescription, you may not kill all the bacteria and you may get sick again. The bacteria that is still alive can then become resistant, making the infection you already have worse, and making it harder to treat.

Cough medicines

Coughing helps your lungs get rid of mucus. Your condition may get worse if you don't cough this up. When you have a wet cough with a lot of thick mucus, your doctor may prescribe a **cough expectorant.** This will help loosen the mucus and make it easier to cough up. It **will not stop you from coughing.**

Tell your doctor if long spells of dry coughing keep you awake at night. He or she may give you a cough suppressant to help you cough less. **Do not take any cough suppressant without asking your doctor.**

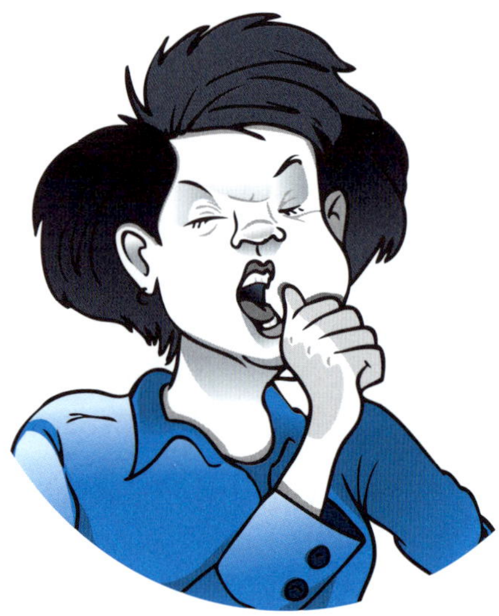

Medications to thin secretions

Keeping your secretions thin makes them easier to cough up. Drinking plenty of water is the best way to keep secretions thin. But sometimes, water is not enough.

– **Guaifenesin** *(Mucinex®, Humibid®)*

This medicine is used to help thin secretions. While this medicine may help, you must still drink plenty of water while taking it.

You don't need a prescription for this and you can get it at your pharmacy. The usual dosage is 1-2 tablets every 12 hours. You may only need this when you have a cold or infection. Or your doctor may want you to take it on a regular basis. Be sure and check with your doctor before taking this or any other medication.

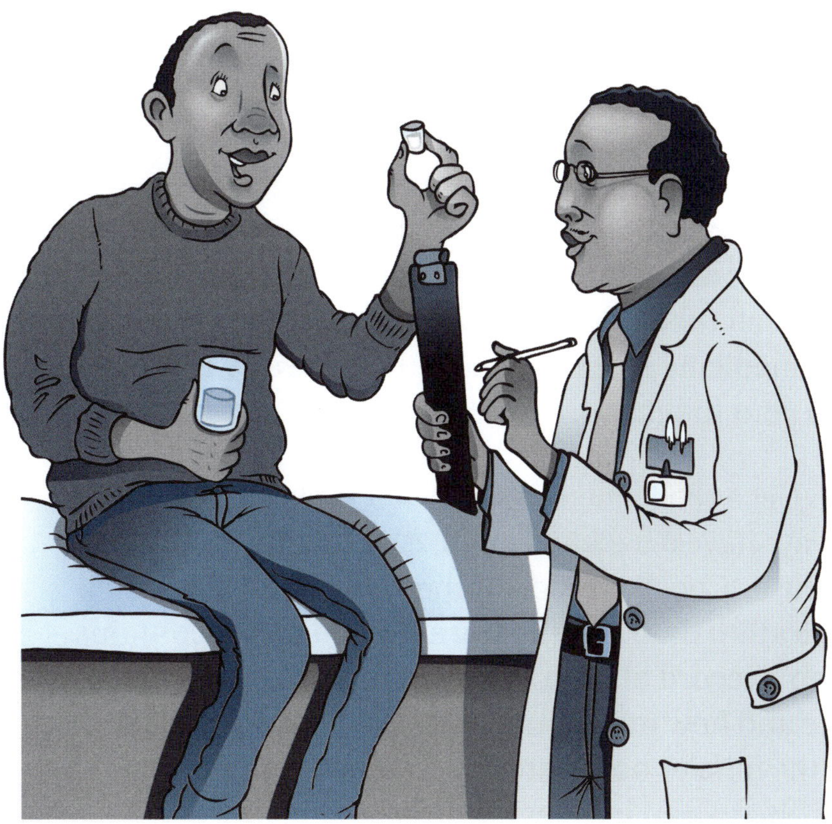

Ways to take medicines

Medicines for COPD can be taken in many ways. They can be taken by liquid or pill, given by shot or inhaled.

Inhaled medicines

There are a number of ways to spray a fine mist of medicine or moisture into your lungs. The most common way to do this is in the home with a nebulizer or with a metered dose inhaler (MDI) with a spacer device.

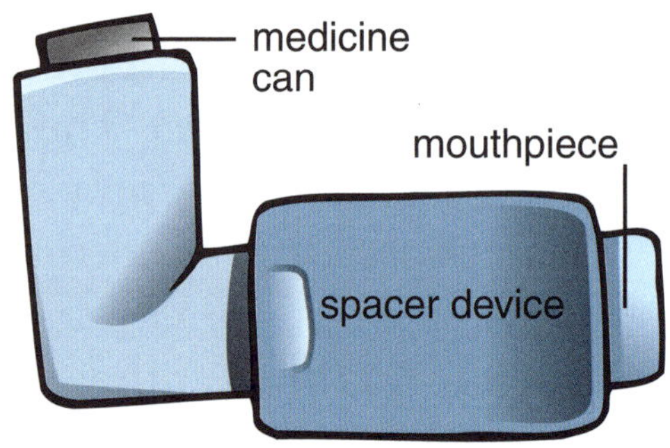

MDI with spacer

The MDI is the easiest and preferred device to use. It is a simple, portable sprayer that is mostly used for inhaling bronchodilators or anti-inflammatory drugs (such as steroids). See the next page for instructions and have your doctor or nurse show you how.

To use the MDI, it is best to use a **spacer device or holding chamber.** Using a spacer makes it easier to get the right amount of medicine to your lungs. One type of spacer is a small tube placed between the MDI and your mouth. The medicine is sprayed into the tube and then inhaled into your lungs.

Get a refill when your inhaler is about 1/4 full. Always have a backup can of each inhaler medicine you use. Check the side of the canister for the **expiration date** and the **number of doses** it contains. **Keep a record** of each dose you use. Write down the date and how many puffs you use, or make a mark on the inhaler box each time you take a puff. You can also use an **inhaler counter** to keep track of doses. You can find this at an asthma and allergy supply center.

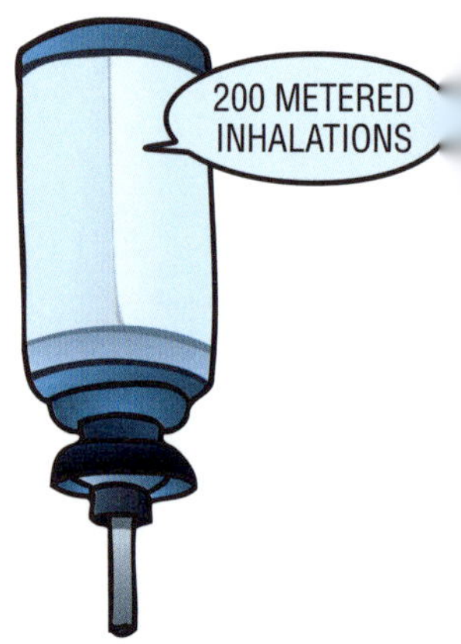

How to use a metered dose inhaler (MDI)

Not all inhalers or spacers are the same. Read the instructions with your package to find out exactly how your inhaler and spacer/holding chamber work. **For all inhalers:**

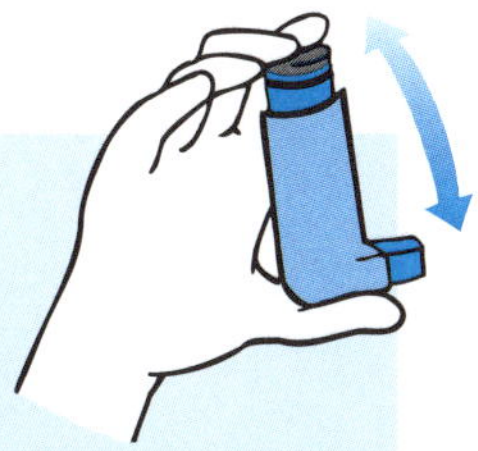

1. Take off the cap. **Shake the inhaler well** before each puff.
2. With the inhaler in the upright position, insert the mouthpiece of the inhaler into the spacer or holding chamber.

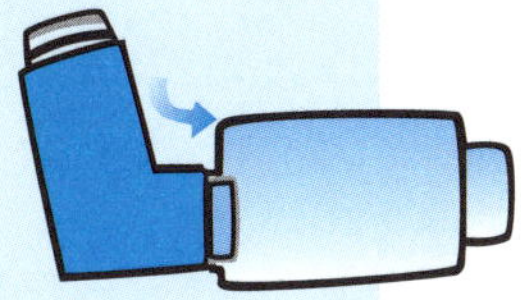

3. Put the mouthpiece of the spacer/holding chamber into your mouth—**over your tongue** and between your teeth. **Seal your lips** around the mouthpiece.

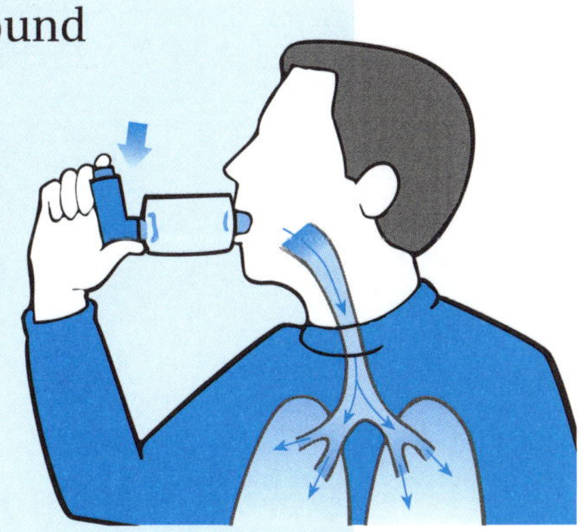

4. Stand up straight. Keep your head level or look up. When ready, gently breathe out.
5. As you start breathing in slowly, press down on the metal can to release 1 puff into the spacer/holding chamber.
6. **Breathe in slowly and deeply** to fill your lungs. **Hold your breath** for 10 seconds.

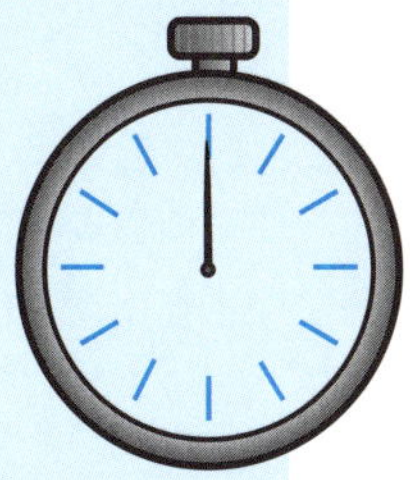

7. If you are supposed to take more than 1 puff, repeat steps 4–6. For the **quick-acting bronchodilators, wait 1 to 2 minutes** between puffs to let the first puff begin working.
8. When you are finished, **rinse** your mouth **and spit.**

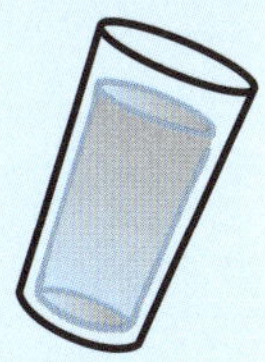

9. Follow the directions on the package to clean and store the inhaler and holding chamber.

CAUTION: The contents of an inhaler are under pressure. Don't keep it or use it near an open flame.

How to use a Diskus® inhaler

Follow these steps when using a Diskus® inhaler:

1. Hold it in one hand and put the thumb of your other hand on the thumbgrip.

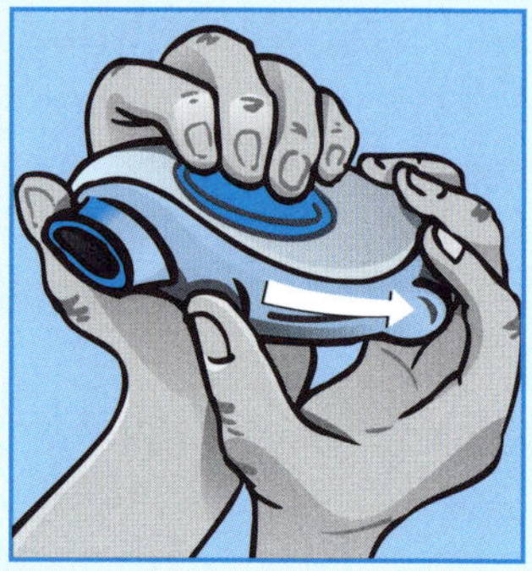

2. Push the thumbgrip away from you until the mouthpiece appears and snaps into place.
3. Hold the inhaler level with the mouthpiece facing you. Put your thumb on the lever and push away from you until it clicks. A dose is now ready.
4. Exhale, but not into the inhaler.

NOTE: Never exhale into the inhaler.

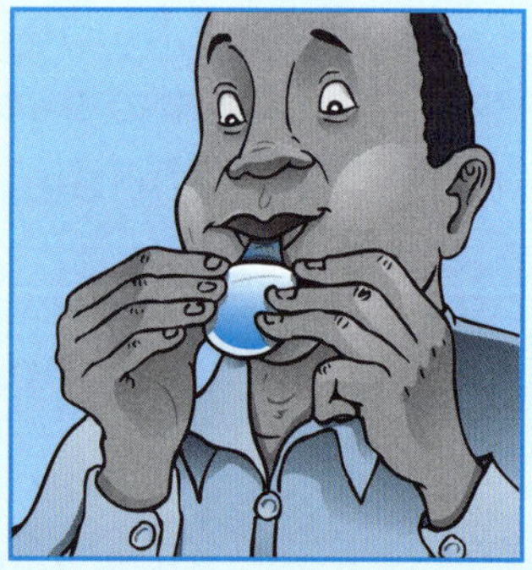

5. Bring the mouthpiece to your lips.
6. Take a quick, deep breath through the inhaler.
7. Hold your breath for 10 seconds.
8. Close the inhaler by sliding the thumbgrip back towards you as far as it will go.
9. Rinse your mouth.

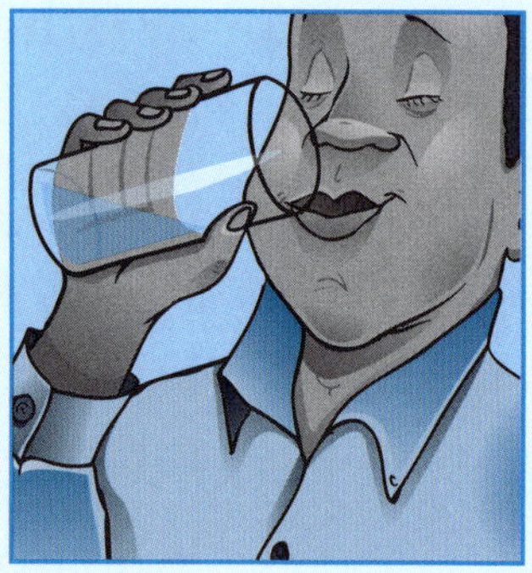

Tips for using the inhaler:

- Always use it in a level position.
- Always keep it dry.
- Rinse your mouth out after every use.
- Never take an extra dose.

Using a HandiHaler®

How to assemble the HandiHaler®:

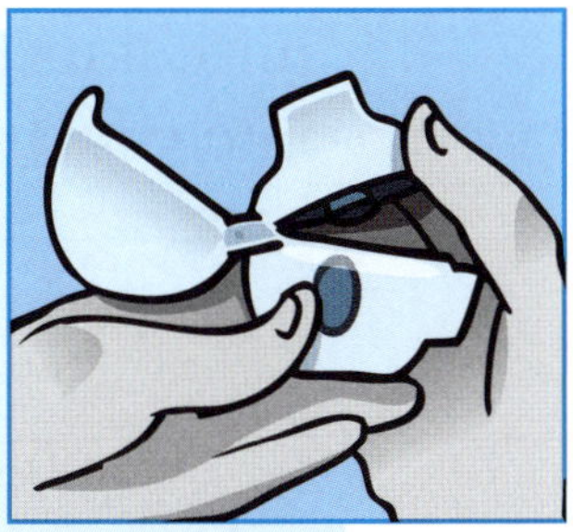

1. Take the capsule out of the blister pack.
2. Open the cover of the HandiHaler®.
3. Open the mouthpiece of the HandiHaler®.
4. Place the capsule in the hole in the center of the HandiHaler®.
5. Close the mouthpiece. You will hear a click.
6. Leave the cover of the HandiHaler® open.

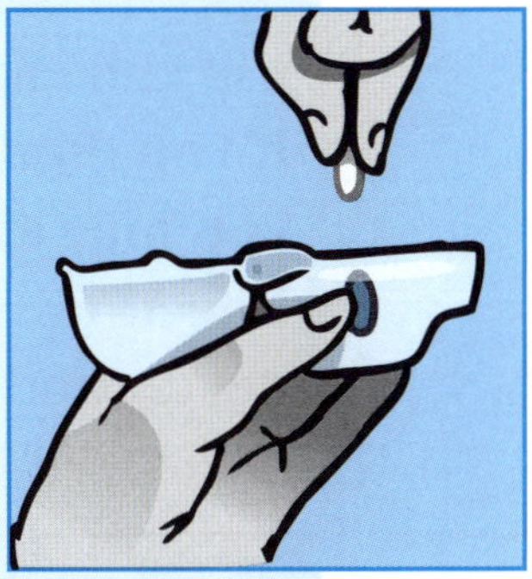

How to use the HandiHaler®:

1. Hold the HandiHaler® with the mouthpiece up. Press the button on the side once to pierce the capsule.
2. With the HandiHaler® away from your mouth, gently breathe out.
3. Seal your lips around the mouthpiece.
4. Inhale slowly and deeply. You should hear the capsule vibrate. Take a full, deep breath.
5. Resume normal breathing.
6. If you did not get in a full breath, repeat steps 2-5 to make sure you breathe in your medicine.
7. Open the mouthpiece and throw away the capsule.

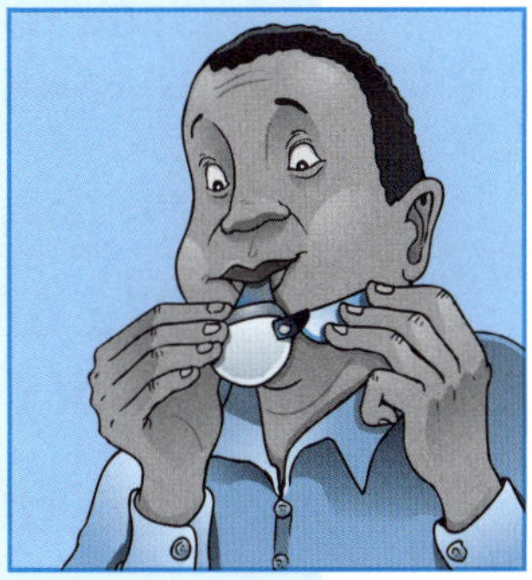

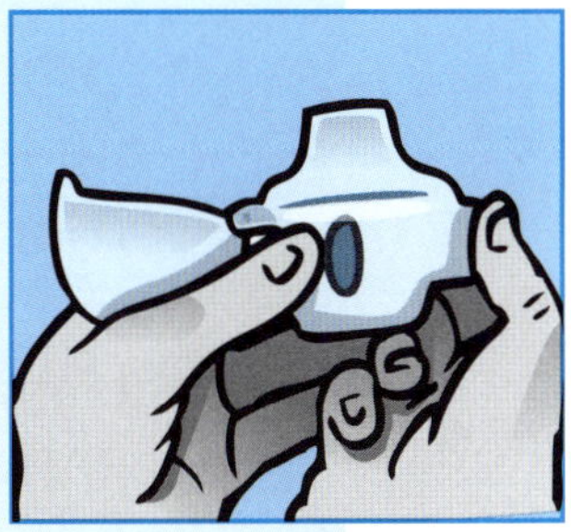

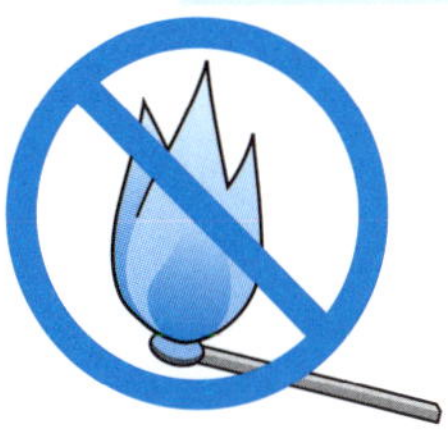

CAUTION: The contents of an inhaler are under pressure. Don't keep it or use it near an open flame.

Using a nebulizer

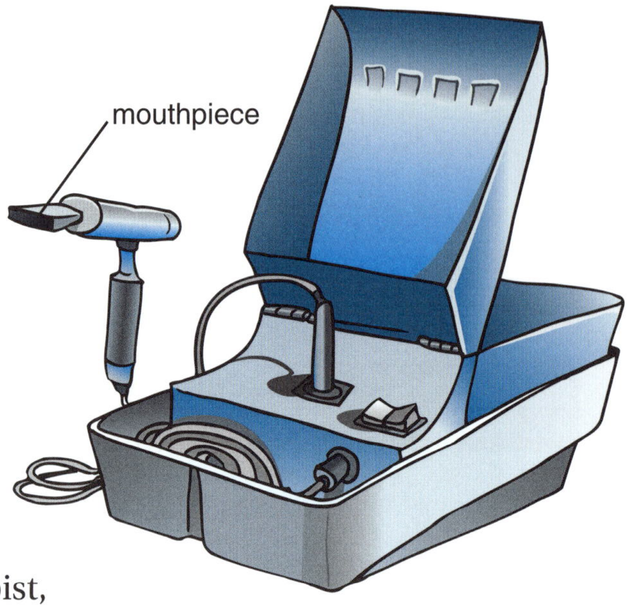

nebulizer

The **nebulizer** sprays a mist of medicine or moisture into your lungs at normal air pressure. It is mostly used for short periods several times a day.

When using a nebulizer, follow your doctor's exact instructions. Know how to use and care for your device. **If you do not clean it properly, you may give yourself a lung infection.** Your respiratory therapist, doctor and the company supplying the device will be able to teach you about its use and cleaning.

The use of any of these devices would be prescribed by your doctor.

The following drugs should only be used on the advice of your doctor:

- **antihistamines or cold medicines** which stop your cough and dry your mucus
- **"water pills"** (diuretics) which are used to rid the body of excess fluid and can also dry your mucus
- **tranquilizers and sedatives** which relax you or help you sleep but can slow your breathing dangerously and interfere with coughing
- **narcotics** which depress breathing and stop coughing

Oxygen

Using oxygen can help you feel better by decreasing shortness of breath, reducing the strain on your heart and enabling you to do regular activities and exercise more easily. If your doctor prescribes oxygen, treat it just like any other medicine. Don't change the amount unless your doctor says to. Your oxygen needs vary with activity. Your oxygen level should be checked at rest, with exercise and when asleep. Your flow rate can then be adjusted to your needs.

The company which provides your oxygen equipment should fully explain its use and care. When your supply arrives, be sure to find out how to reorder. Plan so that you do not run out in the middle of the night or over a weekend or holiday.

To use oxygen safely, do these:

- Store oxygen away from heat or direct sunlight.
- If using cylinders, secure them so that they cannot tip over.
- **No smoking** in the room where oxygen is used or stored.
- **Do not** increase liter flow without asking your doctor.
- **Do not** use any petroleum-based products (such as Vaseline®, certain creams, etc.).
- **Do not** use oxygen near an open flame (such as a gas stove or fireplace).

- You can use electric appliances. But be careful when using things that might spark.

Oxygen Company ______________________________ Phone # __________________

Liter flow at rest ________________ Liter flow with exercise ________________ Liter flow asleep ______________

Hours and/or time of day to use____

Traveling with oxygen

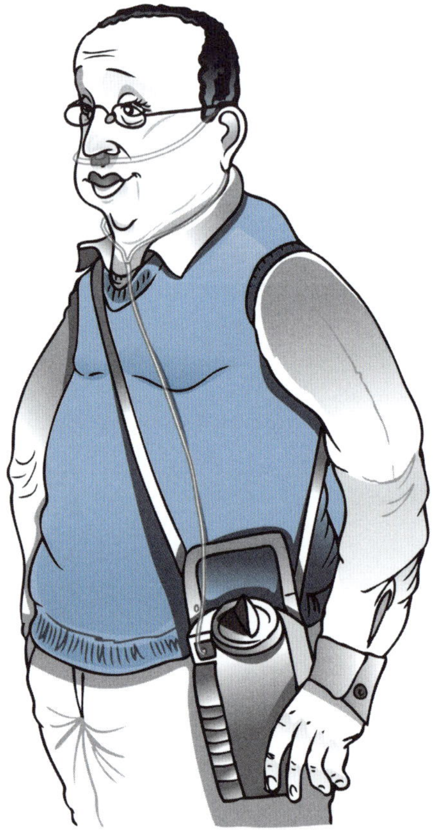

Don't think that being on oxygen means you have to stay home all the time. You can arrange to have oxygen when you travel, whether you go around the corner or around the world! Go to www.portableoxygen.org on the internet for more information.

short trips

Your home care agency or respiratory therapist can set you up for outings of up to 8 or 10 hours. The amount of time depends on tank size and on whether you use liquid or gas oxygen. If you use liquid, it can go in a pack that you carry on your shoulder or wear around your waist. Travel oxygen in gas form comes in a small tank ("E" cylinder) that rolls on wheels or in a smaller tank that can be carried.

longer trips

Ask your oxygen company or home care agency to arrange for your oxygen with a company in the town you plan to visit, or you may make the arrangements yourself.

travel by air

Talk to the airline in advance to see what the rules are for traveling with oxygen. Most airlines will provide it for you because air travel with any type of tank filled with oxygen is unsafe. Just tell the airline your liter flow rate, and they will do the rest. If you have a liquid oxygen system, you may want to take your tank with you to use once you arrive. To do this, just drain the tank dry and leave the top cracked open.

tips for setting up oxygen for a trip

- Know your flow rate.
- If you use a liquid oxygen system, know its brand name. Make sure the new company has the right size adapter to fill your tank.
- Because oxygen is a drug, always take a written prescription with you when you travel.
- Your oxygen supplier can help you with your travel arrangements

For ANY trip, be sure you know:

- how to change tanks when one is empty
- how to measure the amount of oxygen left in your tank
- how to refill your tank (if you have a liquid oxygen system)
- all of the safety measures for oxygen use

❑ Oxygen concentrator

Your doctor may prescribe an oxygen concentrator for you to use. This is an electrical machine that converts the air in your home to almost pure oxygen which you then breathe in through a nasal cannula. Most concentrators also add moisture to the oxygen through a humidifier.

The company that gives you the oxygen concentrator will fully explain how to use and care for it.

Oxygen concentrators are easy to use. They are smaller than the large oxygen tanks. And they don't have to be refilled like liquid oxygen canisters. Some concentrators are even small enough for you to travel with or use in your car.

Even though the oxygen concentrator is easy to use and care for, there are still things you should do to keep it working and keep you safe:

- Keep it clean and free of dust with a damp cloth.
- Replace the nasal cannula (nose tube) about every month.
- Clean the air filter and humidifier (water bottle) every week.
- Do not smoke near it.
- Keep it away from any heat source (space heaters, fireplace, etc.).
- Keep an oxygen tank or liquid oxygen canister as a backup in case the power goes out.
- Keep anything that can catch fire easily (gasoline, alcohol, etc.) away from it.
- If you travel, ask your doctor or nurse about any special plans you need to make before you go.

Chapter 4

Living with COPD

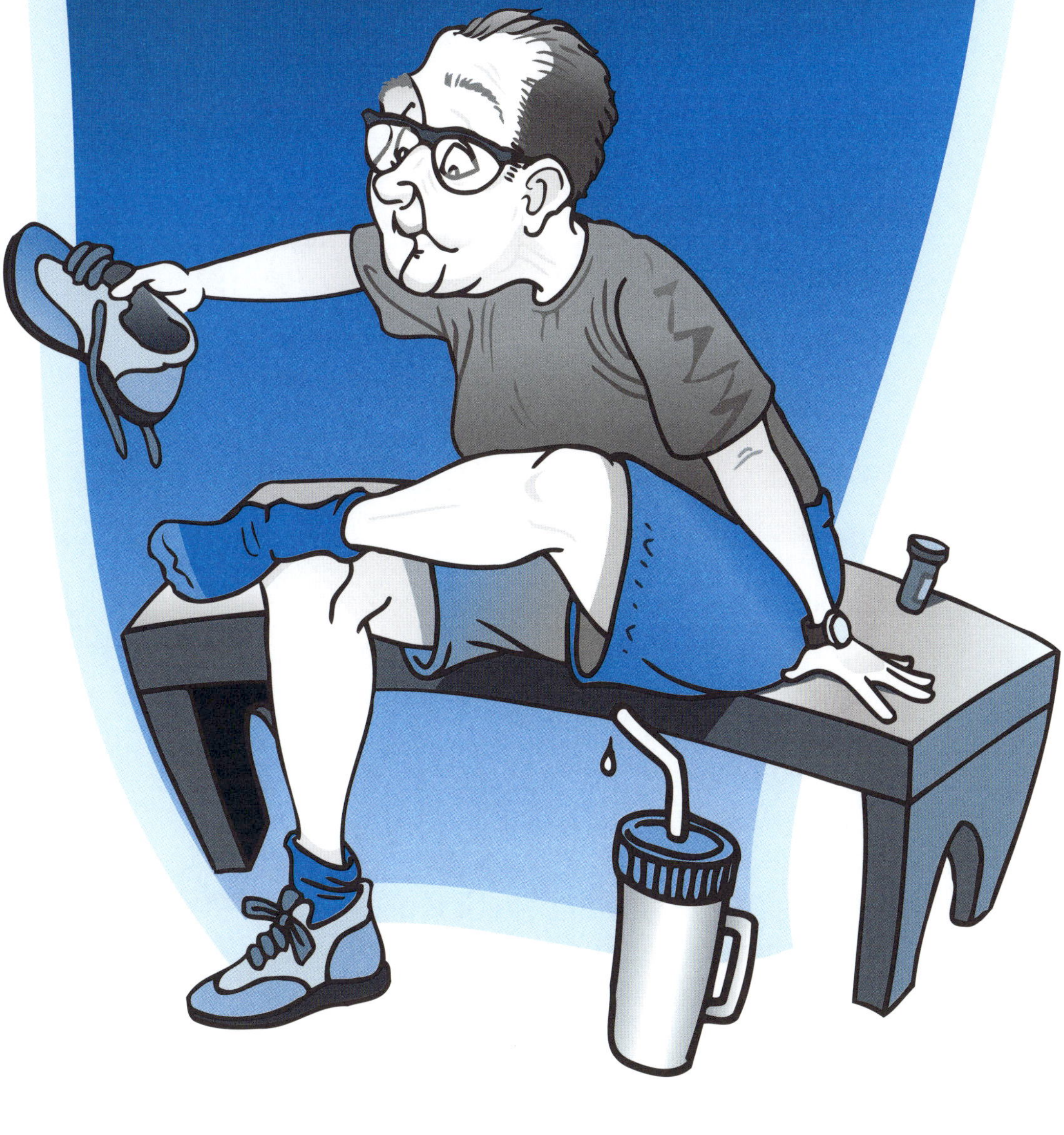

Your emotions

Mood changes can affect how you breathe. Your emotions can cause muscles used for breathing to tighten, making airways narrow and breathing hard. Tense muscles also use more oxygen than relaxed muscles. And when you feel bad, you may not take good care of yourself.

Learning to deal with all kinds of moods will be important to how well you breathe. Lung disease is not fun, and daily treatment can be a real bore. Having someone to talk to helps. Don't try to keep your feelings to yourself. No one can help you if you do.

Here are some of the emotions you may have at one time or another:

- frustration
- anger
- anxiety
- fear
- shock
- disbelief

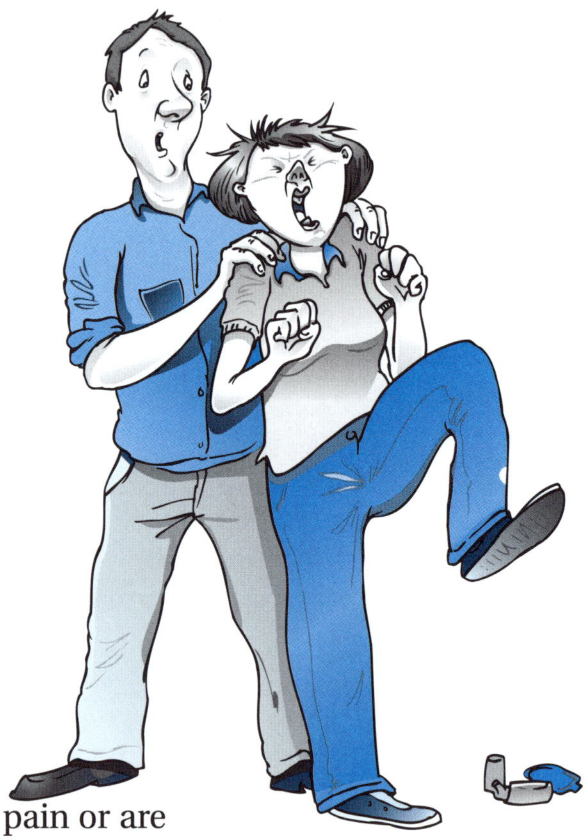

These are all natural responses to living with chronic lung disease. Walking and relaxation or breathing exercises can help a lot. If you stay in pain or are depressed for weeks and nothing helps, talk with your doctor. He or she can help you get back on track and breathe more freely.

Sadness/depression

Sadness or depression can occur when anger is turned inward toward one's self. Feelings of guilt are common, too. Sadness that goes on for a long time can be very painful and harmful. If this happens to you, let your doctor know. It can be treated. Some signs of depression are:

- changes in eating habits
- changes in sleep patterns
- withdrawal from family and friends
- loss of interest in daily activities

There are a number of ways to treat depression. You must find the treatment that's right for you. But there is only one way to know which treatment is best—try it. Some things you can try include:

- talking with a friend, family member or counselor about your feelings
- joining a support group for people with chronic illnesses
- taking an antidepressant medicine (if your doctor prescribes it)
- finding ways to relax and relieve stress—deep breathing, visualizing or mental imagery, or muscle tightening/relaxing
- eating healthy, getting plenty of rest and exercising (as allowed)
- a combination of these

Talk with your doctor about the best treatment for you. Feel free to ask your doctor about possible risks or side effects and the cost of treatment.

Acceptance/control

It takes practice to fit treatment into your daily routine. At times you may feel less in control of your breathing. Don't give up. No one likes having a chronic lung disease, but most learn to accept and live with it. As you adjust to your treatment, your sense of well-being will grow. You will learn to control your lung disease rather than letting it control you.

There are support groups for people with lung disease. One example is the Better Breathers Club. Call the American Lung Association at 1–800–586–4872 for other available resources.

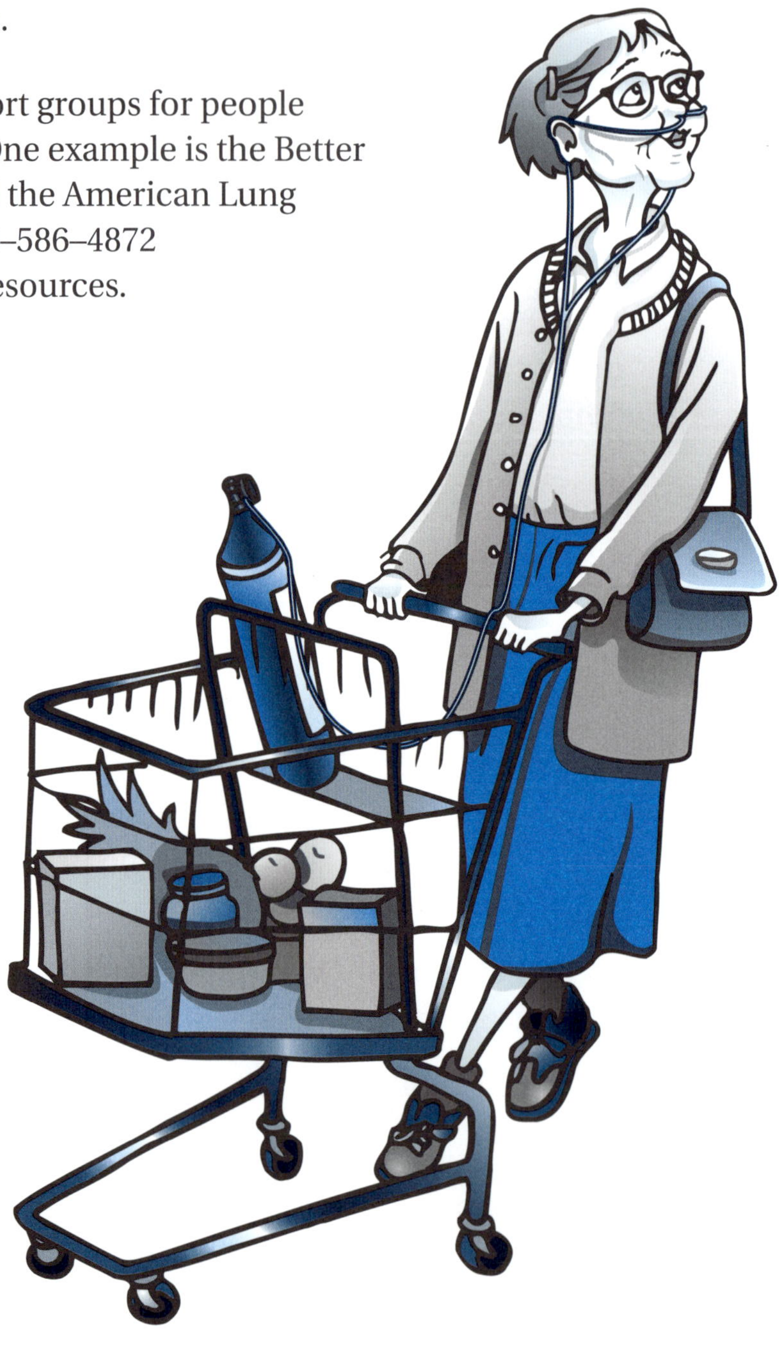

Relaxation exercises

When you relax your body and mind, you reduce muscle tension and relieve anxiety. Use the relaxation steps on the next page to relieve tension when breathing problems increase. The more you practice these, the better you will get at them.

First, find a quiet, peaceful place. Dim the lights, lie down, and put a pillow under your head and knees, or sit up in a straight-backed armchair. Listen to some soft music.

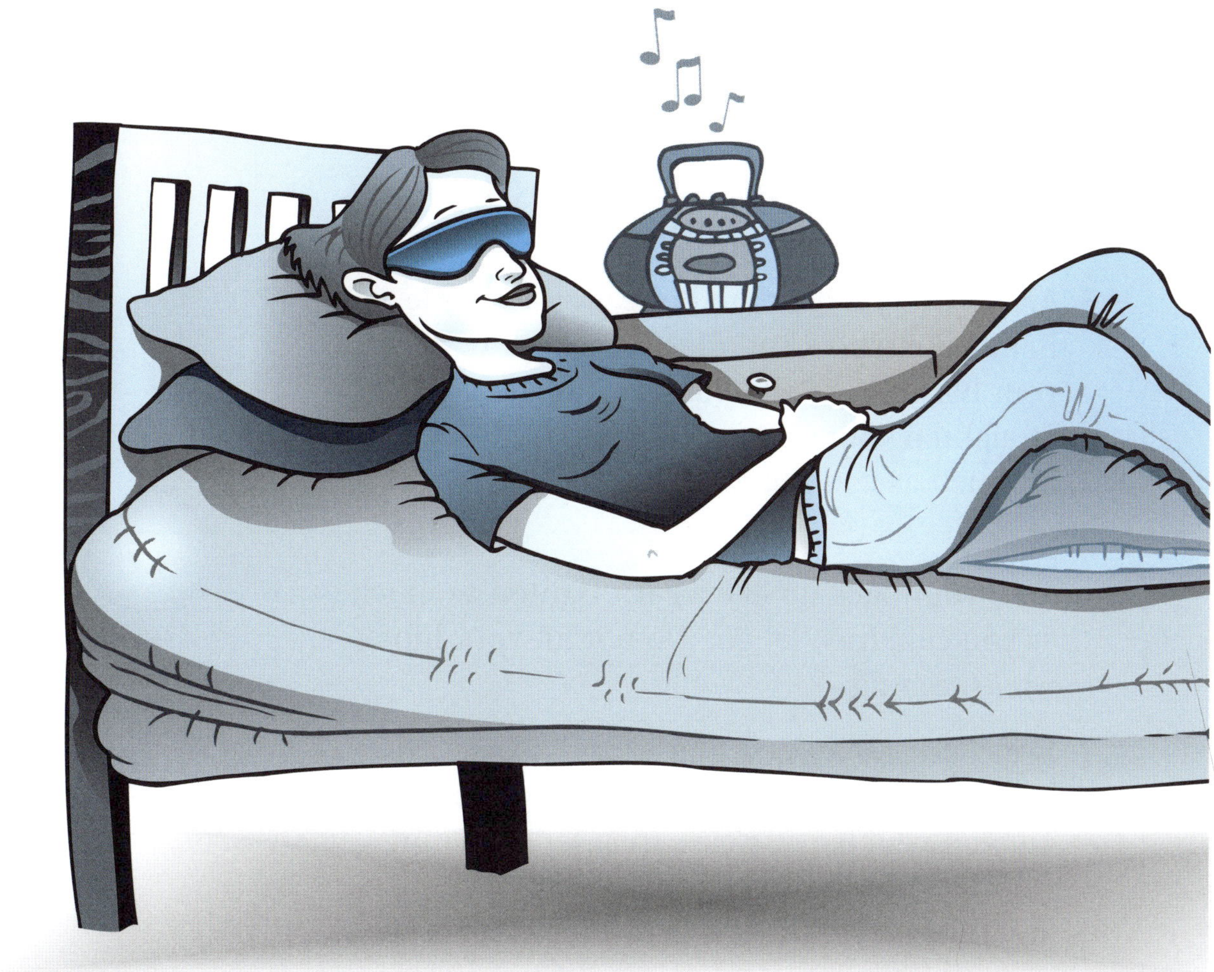

1. **Head and neck**
   Pull your chin down towards your chest as tightly as you can. Then push the back of your head into a pillow. Turn your head from side to side in a relaxed way. Let it stop when it comes to a comfortable position.
2. **Face**
   Tighten ("scrunch") up all of your face muscles. Hold, then let go.
3. **Eyes**
   Focus your eyes on something. Watch it, and slowly let your eyelids grow heavy. Open your eyes, and then let them close slowly until they feel comfortable.
4. **Shoulders**
   Shrug your shoulders and tighten your shoulder muscles. Hold, then let go.
5. **Arms** (Do one hand and one arm at a time.)
   Bend your elbow and make a fist out of your hand. Tighten your fist, then let go. Straighten your arm and fingers. Tighten as much as you can, then let go.
6. **Back**
   Arch your back up like a cat. Tighten as much as you can, then let go. Do not lift your hips while arching.
7. **Legs** (Do one leg at a time.)
   Hold your leg straight and point your toes. Tighten your leg muscles, then let go. Point your toes toward your nose and push your heel and the back of your leg into the bed or floor. Tighten, then let go.

Sex

Having a chronic health problem can upset many parts of a relationship, and this includes sex. But don't write off sex as something you can't enjoy because you have COPD. It is likely that you can function better sexually than you believe.

Start by talking with your partner. Roles and feelings have most likely changed as you and your partner have gotten used to your lung condition. Sharing how each of you feels can renew your relationship and sex life.

Your partner may fear that sex will be too hard on your breathing. Less oxygen in your blood may cause you to feel restless and anxious or on edge. These problems can be solved by time and by talking openly with your partner about the tension, doubts, anger or frustration that either of you have.

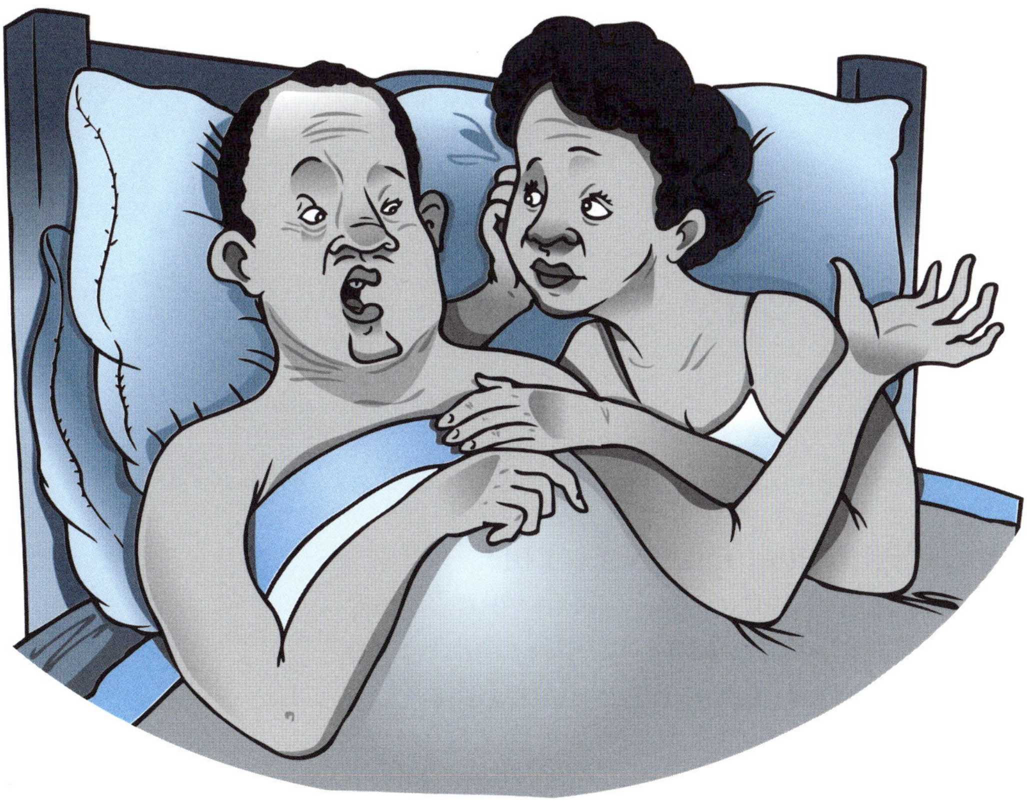

As a person gets older, there are some changes that occur. This is true whether the person has a chronic illness or not. Some of these changes are:

- It takes more time for orgasm to occur.
- There may be a decrease in vaginal lubrication.
- It may take longer to have an erection.
- Some medicines may cause a change in sexual function. If this happens, tell your doctor. He or she may be able to adjust your medicine.

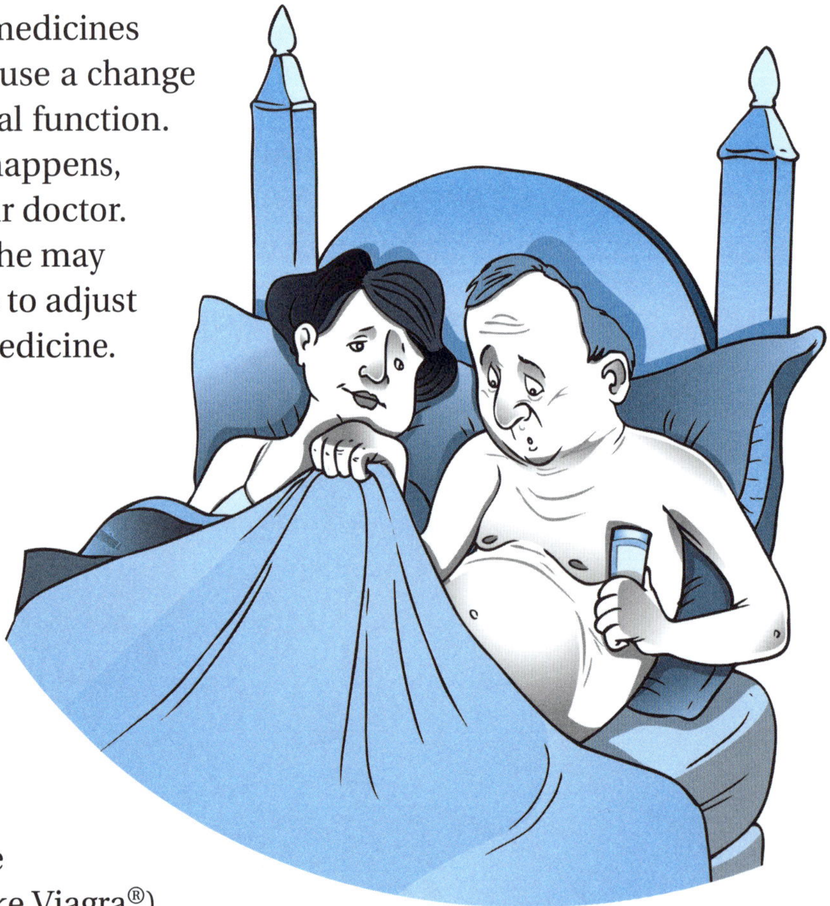

There are medicines (like Viagra®) which may help improve your sex life. If you are interested in one, talk to your doctor about it. **Do not take any over the counter sex aids without talking to your doctor first.**

Better breathing during sex

These may help you breathe more easily during sex:

- Be rested and choose times when breathing is easiest.
- Always wait 2–3 hours after a meal.
- Keep the room cool.
- **Plan to have sex after your bronchodilator has taken effect.**
- During sex, your heart rate and breathing increase. These are normal body changes during sex and are not harmful to you. Use pursed lip breathing to keep your breathing under control.
- If you use oxygen daily, nasal prongs worn during sex will not interfere.
- Don't rush. Give yourself plenty of time to engage in foreplay in a relaxed atmosphere.
- If you start to get anxious, STOP. Relax, cuddle.
- **Make pleasure and affection your goal,** whether you reach orgasm or not.
- Avoid positions that make you support your body on your arms or put added pressure on your stomach. Since you breathe better with your head and chest elevated, you might try these positions:
    - side-lying, either face to face or male behind female
    - female on top—male can recline against the headboard or sit in a chair
    - female sitting with male kneeling or standing
- Keep up your daily breathing and exercise program. A strong body can handle sex better and will help you feel better about yourself and sex.

Air outside and inside

Smoking

If you smoke, find some way to quit. This is the best thing you can do to help control your COPD. Emphysema and chronic bronchitis are most often diseases of smokers. Many things that cause normal cells to change to cancer cells have been found in cigarette smoke. Cigarette smoke also contains nicotine and tar which keep the lungs from cleaning themselves. As a result, dirt particles breathed in from the air get trapped in the lungs. This can lead to infections.

With every puff, you irritate and damage the lining of your lungs. Mucus builds up, the airways swell and the membranes through which oxygen and carbon dioxide are exchanged are destroyed. Then your heart must work harder to pump more blood because your body is crying out for more oxygen. Smoking also increases your heart rate. This can cause you to be more short of breath.

Try not to breathe in second hand smoke either. This is called passive smoking, and it can harm your lungs, too.

No matter how long you have smoked, stopping now will help you breathe better. It will also prevent further damage to your lungs.

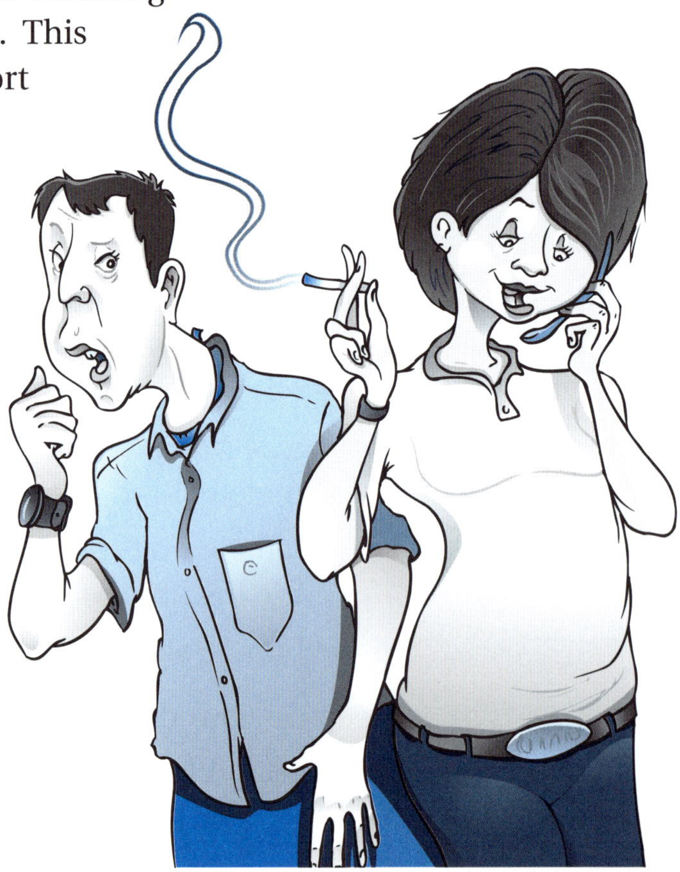

Call your hospital, lung association, clinic or public health nurse to see if there is a stop-smoking or support group to help you quit. Also ask your doctor about inhalers, nasal sprays, medicines or nicotine patches. These products have helped a lot of people stop smoking. Here are some other tips to help you kick the habit:

- Keep your mind active—read a good book, do a jigsaw puzzle or write a letter.
- Find ways to keep your hands busy (like playing with a rubber band, pencil or sponge ball).
- Nibble on healthy snacks, such as carrots, grapes or bread sticks.
- Find ways to relax—take a bath or listen to soft music.
- Change your routines and patterns so that you're less tempted to smoke when you normally would have.
- If you smoked after meals, leave the table as soon as you finish eating and brush your teeth or eat a mint.
- If you smoked in your car, clean it out, and remove the ashtray and lighter.

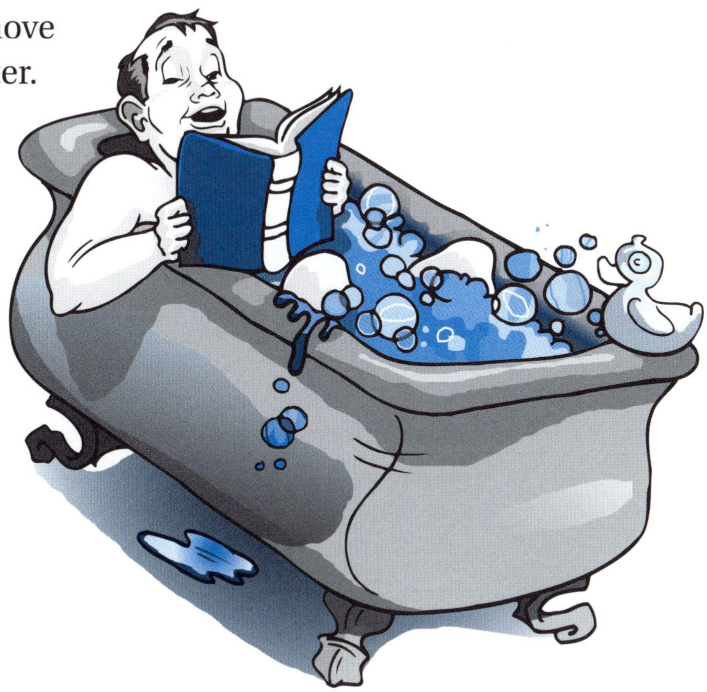

Don't give up if it takes more than one try to quit smoking. **Keep trying.** You can win this battle with your smoking habit.

Pollution

In places where the air is polluted, more people have chronic bronchitis and emphysema. If you can, stay inside a centrally heated or air-conditioned building on days when the pollution count is high (100°F/37.8°C or above).* Always avoid being exposed to air pollution when you can.

Keep your heating and air-conditioning system in good working order. Change filters often.

Weather

Breathing in very cold air can make you cough and wheeze. Breathe through a handkerchief or scarf to warm the air before it hits your lungs. You can also buy **cold weather masks.**

Either a humid or dry climate can be a problem. An air-conditioner or a dehumidifier can dry out air that is too damp. A humidifier can be used to moisten air that is too dry. (Dry air is often a problem in winter when the heat is on.) A humidifier can also be used to settle dust. **Clean all humidifiers often.**

You may have to try it out to see whether a damp or dry climate suits you best. A humidity level of 40–50% is most often the best for easy breathing.

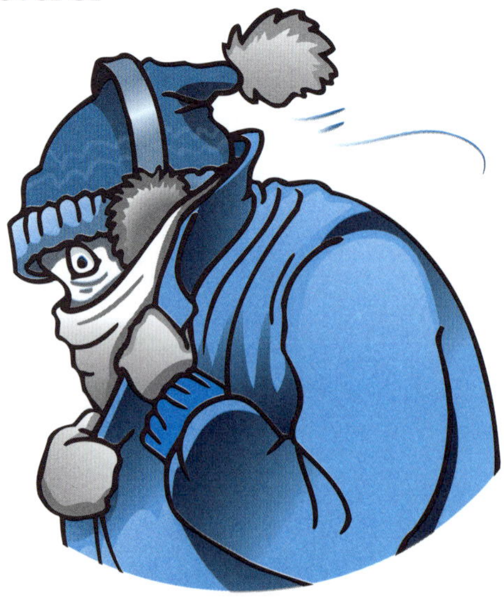

** You can often find what the pollution count (index) is by calling weather information at your local TV station. This count is sometimes given as part of the weather update on the news.*

Household fumes

Avoid strong fumes from cleaning products and use a venting fan over the stove to get rid of cooking fumes. Use products which are poured or rubbed instead of those in spray cans. Sprayed fumes are easy to inhale.

Dust

Dust-raising jobs in your house or yard can make it harder for you to breathe. If you must do a "dusty" job, wear a handkerchief, dust mask or filter over your mouth and nose. Best of all, have someone else dust your house when you aren't home. Stay away from your house for at least 45 minutes after it has been cleaned and dusted.

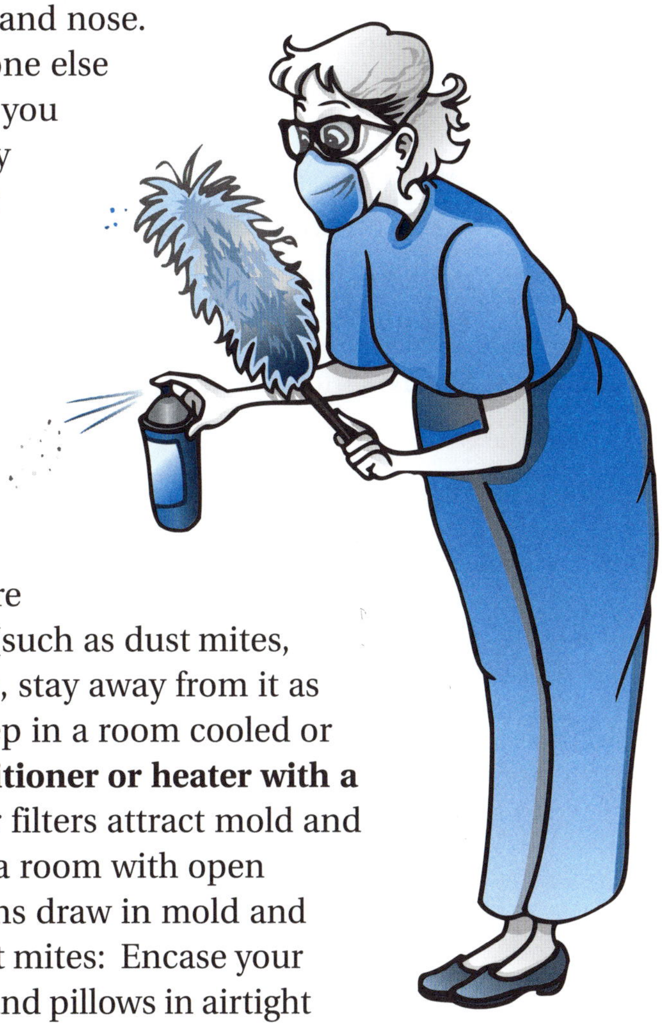

Allergies

If you know you are **allergic** to something (such as dust mites, cats, dogs, grass, trees), stay away from it as much as you can. Sleep in a room cooled or heated by an **air-conditioner or heater with a CLEAN filter.** Dirty air filters attract mold and germs. Don't sleep in a room with open windows and fans. Fans draw in mold and pollen. To control dust mites: Encase your bed mattress, springs and pillows in airtight vinyl covers. Wash all bedding in hot water. Don't put carpet on your bedroom floor. Your doctor will suggest medicine or allergy shots if you need them.

Foods*

Choose foods with care. You need to eat foods from all the food groups and drink a lot of fluid. Your diet has a direct effect on how healthy you are and how well your body can fight off infections. Choosing your meals from the food groups shown here will help keep your body as strong and healthy as possible.

- **Grains** – includes all foods made from wheat, rice, oats, cornmeal or barley. At least half of all grains eaten should be whole grains.
- **Vegetables** – includes all fresh, frozen, canned or dried vegetables and vegetable juices. Vegetables are sub-divided into dark green, orange, legumes (beans), starches and all others. A variety of vegetable types should be eaten each week. Fresh or frozen vegetables are best, if your diet limits your sodium (salt) intake. Canned vegetables have more sodium in them.
- **Fruits** – includes all fresh, frozen, canned or dried fruits and fruit juices.
- **Oils** – includes fats from many different plants and fish. Fats that are liquid at room temperature include canola, corn, olive, soybean and sunflower oil. Some foods are naturally high in oils, like nuts, olives, fish and avocados. Some processed foods are mainly oil, such as mayonnaise, some salad dressings and soft margarine. Some plant oils, such as coconut and palm kernel, are high in saturated fat and should be avoided.
- **Milk** – includes all fluid milk products, yogurt and cheese. Other foods made from milk, like cream cheese, cream and butter, are not part of the group (they have little to no calcium in them).
- **Meat and Beans** – includes 1 oz of lean meat, poultry or fish, 1 egg, 1 tablespoon (Tbsp) peanut butter, ¼ cup cooked dry beans or ½ ounce (oz) of nuts or seeds (equal to 1 oz of meat or beans).

** This information is not for use by CF patients who must follow a very special diet.*

The food pyramid can help you to create a custom-made meal plan. How much you eat of each of the 6 groups is based on your age, sex and level of activity. Visit www.mypyramid.gov for more information.

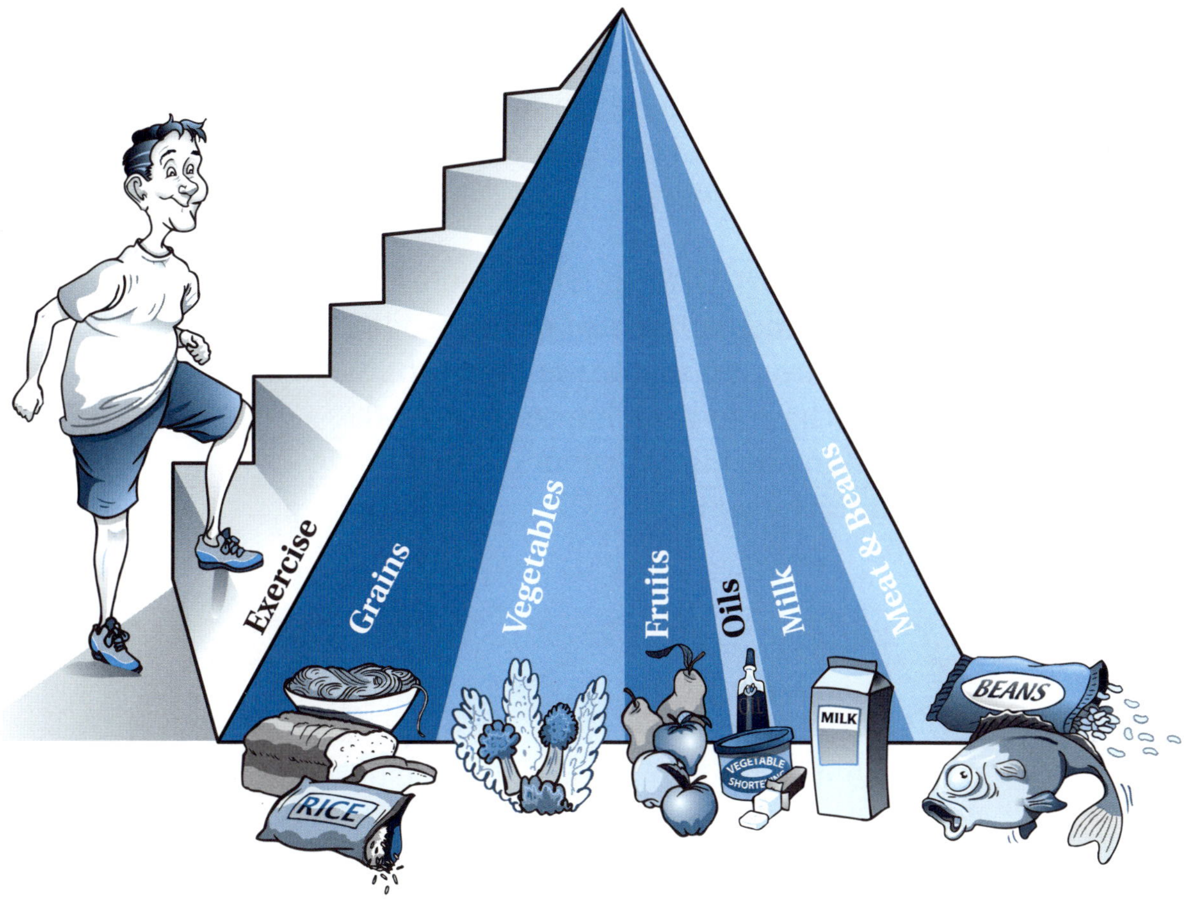

Even if you've been following the same diet for years, you may notice that you've been losing weight. This is because your body works a little harder to breathe. So, the number of calories you need may be slightly different for you. Ask your doctor, nurse or dietitian about a diet to best suit your needs.

Drink 8-16 cups of water and other liquids (including milk) each day.*

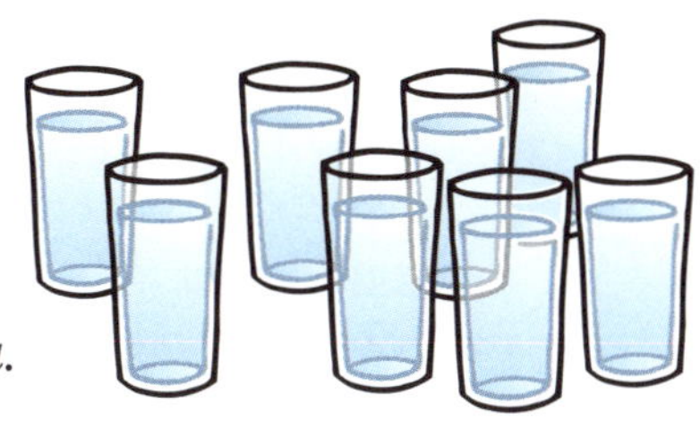

** Ask your doctor if 8-16 cups of fluid is OK for you. Some people can't drink a lot of fluids because of kidney disease, prostate trouble or heart disease.*

If you are too thin and need to gain weight, the quickest way to add calories is by eating more healthy foods during the day (5–6 small meals) and by not skipping meals. Try to eat more fruits and vegetables, lean cuts of meat, and breads or pastas.

You can also ask your doctor about taking nutritional supplements. These are sold at most grocery and drug stores and can give you extra calories, vitamins and minerals.

Some people with COPD should avoid a lot of sweets, desserts and carbonated drinks (soda). These produce more carbon dioxide than other foods. The lungs have to work harder to get rid of the extra carbon dioxide. Ask your doctor if this is a problem for you.

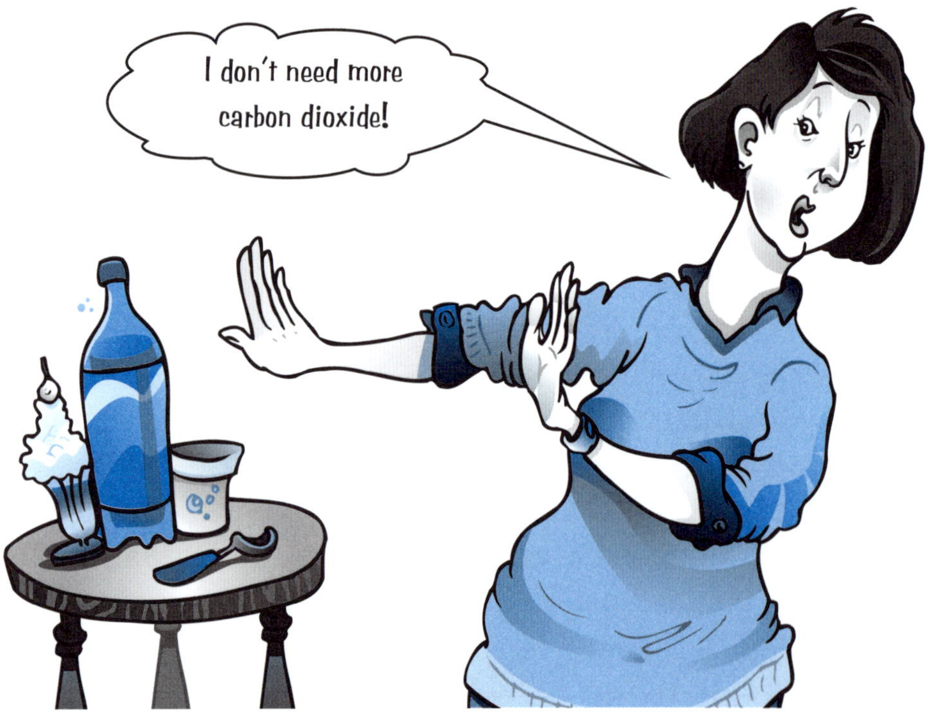

** Ask your doctor if 8–16 cups of fluid a day is OK for you. Some people can't drink a lot of fluids because of kidney disease, prostate trouble or heart disease.*

How much you eat at one time can affect your breathing. Eating a large meal can leave you feeling too full and short of breath. Eating 5–6 smaller meals and 3 snacks each day will make the stomach less full. This leaves more room for your lungs to expand when you breathe. Another way to avoid that "too full" feeling is to eat less of the foods that cause gas. If the foods on this list bother you, eat less of them or use some kind of anti-gas medicine to relieve your symptoms.

- apples (raw)
- asparagus
- beans (pinto, kidney, black, navy)
- broccoli
- brussels sprouts
- cabbage
- carbonated drinks
- cauliflower
- corn
- cucumbers
- melons
- onions (raw)
- peas (split, blackeye)
- peppers
- pimientos
- radishes
- rutabagas
- turnips

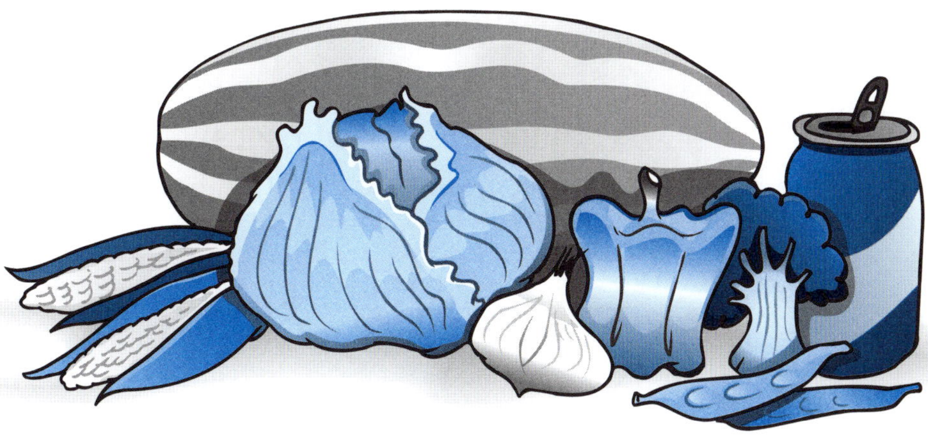

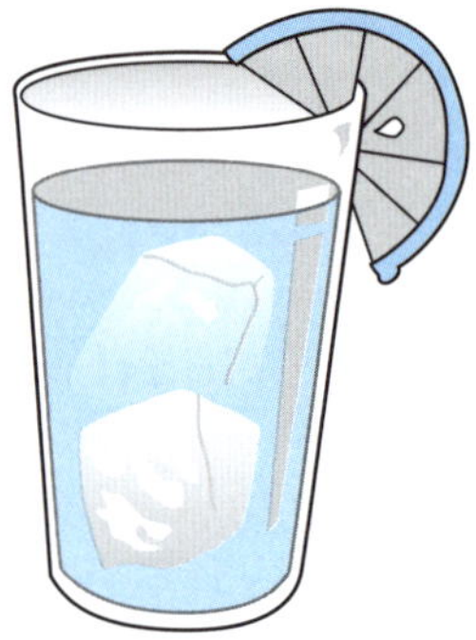

There may be days when you feel very stopped up with mucus. On these days, highly acidic drinks like **lemonade or orange juice** may help control the mucus in your throat.

Some people with COPD think that drinking milk causes increased mucus or breathing trouble. Milk does not make mucus thicker. But it may coat the back of your throat and make it feel thicker. Rinsing your mouth with water after drinking milk will prevent this problem.

If you don't drink milk, you can get calcium and protein by eating cheese, sardines with bones, green leafy vegetables, eggs and meat. Some antacids (like Tums® or Rolaids®) are a good source of calcium. Ask your doctor what kind and how much extra calcium you should take (if any).

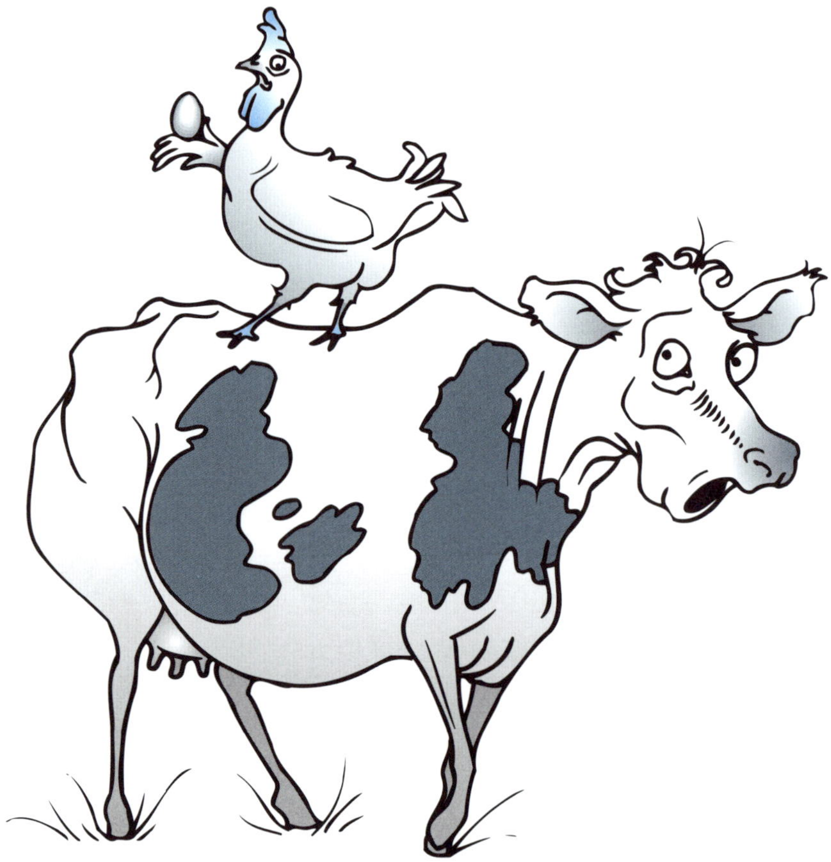

Weight tracking

It is important for you to keep track of your weight so you will know if your body is retaining fluid. You can do this by using the chart below to record your weight each day.

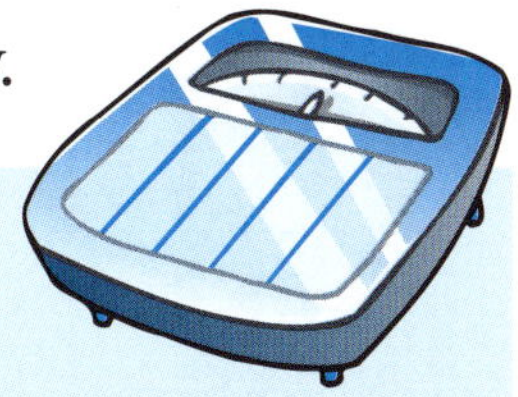

My normal body weight range is: __________ - __________
(Ask your doctor or nurse to tell you these numbers.)

Notes: ____

____

Date/Time	Weight

Date/Time	Weight

Ask your doctor to help you fill in this chart.

______________________'s Medicine Chart

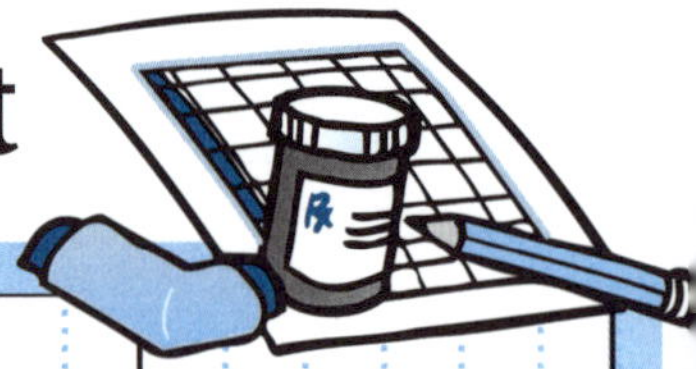

Name	Type	What it does	When to take	How to take	How long to take	When you will feel it working	What to do if you for-get to take	Side effects and what to do about them

This page may be copied for your use.

Ask your doctor to help you fill in this chart.

________________'s Treatment Plan

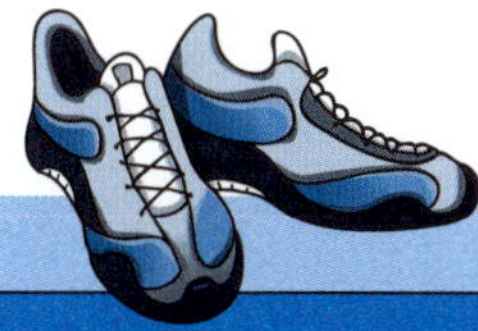

Treatment	See page(s)...	Details (how often, how long, etc.)
❑ Pursed lip breathing	6–7	
❑ Diaphragmatic breathing	20–22	
❑ Controlled coughing	9–10	
❑ Water drinking	11–12	
❑ Aerobic exercise	17–18	
❑ Breathing exercises	19–24	
❑ Diet	72–76	
❑ Weight tracking	77	
❑ Medicines	38–58 78	see medicine chart
❑ Other		

Final notes

Use what you have learned in this book and from other sources and stick to your treatment each day. While taking care of your lungs, do these:

- Ask your doctor, nurse, respiratory therapist or physical therapist any questions you may have.
- Drink lots of fluids each day (unless not allowed for other health reasons).
- Take the drugs prescribed for you.
- Make breathing and body exercises a daily habit.
- Eat foods that will keep you healthy and help you fight infection.
- Talk with your family about the changes made in your life by COPD.
- Choose a goal and work toward reaching it.
- Get involved in a pulmonary rehab program or support group for lung disease.

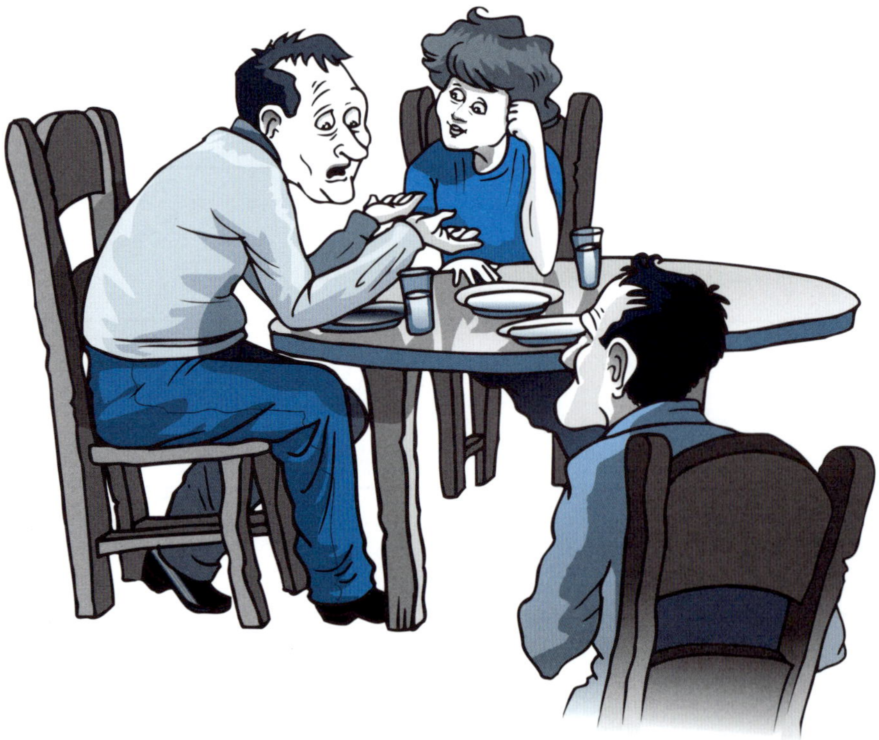